MW00843723

Both/And

Medicine and Public Health Together

by

Katie Kaney, DrPH, MBA, FACHE

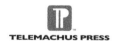

TELEMACHUS PRESS

Both/And——Medicine and Public Health Together
Copyright © 2023 by Katie Kaney, DrPH, MBA, FACHE. All rights reserved, including the right to reproduce this book, or portions thereof, in any form. No part of this text may be reproduced, transmitted, downloaded, decompiled, reverse engineered, or stored in or introduced into any information storage and retrieval system, in any form or by any means, whether electronic or mechanical without the express written permission of the author. The scanning, uploading, and distribution of this book via the Internet or via any other means without the permission of the publisher is illegal and punishable by law. Please purchase only authorized electronic editions and do not participate in or encourage electronic piracy of copyrighted materials.

The publisher does not have any control over and does not assume any responsibility for author or third-party websites or their content.

Cover design byTelemachus Press, LLC

Cover art:
Copyright© Shutterstock/1096542335/sadedesign

Whole Person Index and graphic are trademarks of Katie Kaney and Patent Pending.

Publishing Services by Telemachus Press, LLC
7652 Sawmill Road Suite 304
Dublin, Ohio 43016
http://www.telemachuspress.com

ISBN# 978-1-956867-50-3 (eBook)
ISBN# 978-1-956867-51-0 (Paperback)

Library of Congress Control Number: 2022921779

Version 2023.01.30

Acknowledgements/Contributors

It is an honor and a privilege to share these pages with the extraordinary leaders showing us the way. My deepest gratitude and respect for each person listed below. Real change happens in teams, supporting each other. Let's go.

Forward by **J. Lloyd Michener, MD, FAAFP**

Real-World Population Health Analytics in Community, Public, and Medical Health Systems
Ines M. Vigil, MD, MPH, MBA
Martha L. Sylvia PhD, MBA, RN

Convergence of Diagnostics and Population Health: Clinical Lab 2.0
Khosrow R. Shotorbani, MBA, MT
KathleenM. Swanson, MS, RPh
Mark K Fung, MD, PhD
Jill Warrington, MD, PhD
Beth Bailey
Michael J Crossey, MD, PhD

Editor **Elizabeth Wagner**

Publisher **Steve Himes**

OUTLINE OF CONTENTS

Both/And

Medicine and Public Health Together

Foreword

INTEGRATING MEDICINE AND public health has been a topic in the United States for decades, but until recently this integration has lacked a driving force that could realign roles and relationships and demonstrate the value of partnerships. COVID-19 and the growing awareness of systemic racism has changed the dynamic, highlighting the absence of trust between many community members and public health organizations as well as the value of partnerships between communities, healthcare groups, and public health. Now, as healthcare systems and practitioners grapple with new attention to variation in health outcomes by race, ethnicity, gender, sexual orientation, social class, and location, it has become clear that healthcare groups alone cannot effectively address systemic barriers to health equity. But we can be key partners in broader community-based coalitions for health, working together to improve the communities where people live, work, and play.

For clinicians, the transition from being the respected expert in the exam room or hospital to one of many advisors to community groups, who may not always place healthcare at the top of their concerns, can be challenging, humbling, and ultimately inspiring. This book by Katie Kaney and colleagues will ease that transition, providing facts, figures, and new ways of thinking about health, healthcare, and public health, along with stories and examples that illuminate the path ahead. Equally important, Dr. Kaney and team call out some of the lessons learned, so that those new to this work can avoid efforts that medicalize social needs, engage healthcare teams in efforts far from their capacity, or add untenable new workloads to already overloaded healthcare groups. We may still be early in the stages of learning about effective partnerships between medicine and public health, but we have learned a lot about what not to do and have found examples of successful approaches such as those shared here.

Of all the lessons learned, perhaps the most important is that medicine and public health really can work together, with community partners, sharing data and collaborating on community-led projects that weave together the threads of our diverse communities, and improve health and health equity. The journey to improve health has been long and costly, but it is finally gathering momentum, and we may finally be able to see our children and our neighbors live longer and healthier lives than our own. This book is an important part of the movement to healthy and resilient people in all communities, and a source of ideas and inspiration for the work yet to be done.

J. Lloyd Michener, MD, FAAFP
Editor, *The Practical Playbook I, II,* and *III*

Introduction
Together: Medicine and
Public Health

Questions for a New Day

IMAGINE IF WE systemically joined the care of the individual to the care of the community. What would that look like? We know that the health of the community is public health and the health of the individual is medicine, but are those professions aligned in our current system? Do they work together effectively? Would effective alignment even be possible? What would it look like? Could now be the time to answer these questions?

Our health is constructed of our individual makeup and choices AND the circumstances and communities in which we live.

While our systems often silo the treatment of the individual as something separate from community efforts, we can't escape the interaction between these two. All factors drive our ultimate health. The existing work focused on the community and the individual needs to be purposefully integrated if we are going to get better results.

This is not a new topic. However, it's a new day. At least, it could be a new day, if we truly take advantage of the opportunities a global pandemic has presented us: forced acknowledgement of the interdependence of public health and medicine, funding, public expectations, and, most importantly, the restlessness of those in the health and healthcare professions to make the changes needed to the traditional system to get better results.

The Journey

Let's go on this journey together. The research and evidence show the benefits of joining the care of the individual to the care of the community—**why haven't we done it?**

To those who read this and say we have, I don't disagree: we have in some cases, and we are talking about the opportunities more than ever. However, we need to ask ourselves—does our system of health and healthcare currently align incentives and support the integration of public health and medicine? Does the system inherently ensure the gifts of both public health and medicine are applied *first* and then

> **... does our system of health and healthcare currently align incentives and support the integration of public health and medicine?**

a critical business eye ensuring a measurable return on investment (ROI), to fully realize its potential? Or is the opportunity for the moment being squandered in silos? Or wasted because of money? Or business justifications? Do we see public health trying to advance programs to address social determinants but not the overall system? Do we see medicine striving for incremental change focused on equity but not looking beyond the traditional utilization model of sick care? Do we see community organizations duplicating missions to fill the gaps? Do we see payers prioritizing prevention but preserving net margins? Do we recognize that all of this is happening without sharing data and insights to prioritize, measure, and continuously and reliably improve the output of the health system for all?

Poor Health Costs All of Us

We fundamentally have to prove the ROI of health. Business and financial acumen is essential to apply to the implementation of health. It is the critical ingredient after the science is understood. However, we cannot start or end with the business proposition— the business application and value are just one part of the process. Too often the business rigor is applied before the longitudinal impact of the

The question is not is there enough money, but what it is spent on, what outcomes it drives, and what outcomes we are satisfied achieving together.

health issue is understood. This causes, at best, fragmentation, lack of alignment, and episodic solutions/ treatments. At worst, we build systems which inherently foster inequity, false prioritization, and the application of tools that are not compatible to address the root causes. Our system should incentivize a combination of acute AND preventive solutions reliably applied to the population and individual based upon the data which shows their impact across diverse individuals and populations.

The pot of money being spent on health and health care is abundant. The question is not is there enough money, but what it is spent on, what outcomes it drives, and what outcomes we are satisfied achieving together.

Healthcare Pitfalls with Public Health Solutions

Digging deeper into healthcare, there are elements of prevention and public health woven in the American system. However, the tools and treatments from a medical acumen are "prescribed" much more frequently and confidently than the tools of public health. Pediatrics, for example, bases the medical approach to the health and wellness of kids with its inclusion of well checks, immunizations, and health behavior assessments built into the expectations. The system supports it as well, only allowing children to attend school with proper immunizations (yes, we already have a vaccine mandate for all Americans and have for decades). The problem is, unfortunately, once you age out of the "well child" checks, the traditional healthcare system does not proactively care about you until you get pregnant, have a chronic disease (unlikely for most until their mid 40s), or age into your next wave of prevention (for example, mammograms and colonoscopies). What system is supporting health during the years post childhood? Or in underserved areas without adequate access to childhood healthcare, what options are in place? Some may answer it's an individual's responsibility.

Some answer the employer has stepped in to serve the role. Others say the payer is the gateway or keeper to health. All of these answers are correct. The larger question could be what is the ease of health for people across America including access to healthcare and public health solutions? Do we know? Is it measured?

Using myself as an example, I would often joke during my time as a healthcare executive that the broader "system" cared about me a lot when I was a geriatric pregnant person at 40 and needed my mammogram. I suddenly was contacted and sought after. Until then, all of the healthcare or health I received from ages 18 to 40 was largely driven if I chose to go see the physician for my annual checkup (and the dentist and optometrist) or needed to seek care because of sickness or an acute episode. I was fortunate to have access to such, including insurance coverage, but, even if you have this access, during the 20 years between your end of run with the pediatrician and your aging into chronic illness, you are almost a nobody to the traditional healthcare system—unless you are sick. This is changing some with the rise of consumerism in health.

If you are one of many who have never had access to a pediatrician or a primary care provider or a dentist, then, for you, this journey began almost from birth (and even prior to that, if you look at infant mortality rates in our country) and consists of the safety net primary care solution of the emergency department (ED). This makes many people upset: the number of people who seek primary care in the ED. But, I have always countered that this is exactly the system healthcare has set up, so why are we upset about it?

Using data and analytics, the prominence of primary care offices in affluent zip codes far surpasses that of lower socio-economic areas. If you don't have convenient access or education or insurance to go to a primary care doctor or a dentist, the only other option provided is the ED. When people are not made aware of their options, and not given the power of knowledge, they are unable to make an informed decision. The patient's trust also has to be earned by the healthcare system. The most effective efforts are built from the community voice—out ensuring the approach and solutions take into account local dynamics and cultures partnered with experts in healthcare and public health.

Public Health Problems with Healthcare Consequences

Food insecurity is another powerful example of our systemic problems. Food insecurity is a solvable problem. Hunger is a distribution issue, not a supply issue. We have plenty of food—healthy food. But it is maldistributed. As in the example above about lack of access to primary care, the system is built to drive the exact outcomes it is designed to produce. Because of a dependence on data and analytics, grocery chains are not necessarily building stores in low socio-economic neighborhoods. The food available in these neighborhoods is often fast food restaurants or convenience stores with little to no fresh food.

In the same way that the healthcare system has tried to solve the primary care access problem for children, the federal government and public health partners have tried to address the problem of food insecurity. One solution is the National

School Lunch Program creating access to food through the education system since 1946 [1]. Another is the Supplemental Nutrition Assistance Program (SNAP) program which provides food purchasing assistance to qualifying families and individuals. Other key nongovernmental programs such as Feed America, Meals on Wheels, pantry systems, community gardens, etc., fill in the gaps to help solve the distribution issue. Increasingly, solutions are incorporating technology and at home-food delivery [2].

Back in the late 2000, I recall attending an American College of Healthcare Executives conference in Chicago. One of the topics featured a speaker from the Food and Drug Administration (FDA) speaking about the SNAP program and its clinical value to patients. I don't remember the exact figures, but I also remember learning about how this money was earmarked to help provide options for people to pay for food (hopefully healthy) so if it was not spent for food, it was not used. The statistic they shared about the high percentage of returned funds (double digits) was very impactful to me. And to the other four people who attended the session. Of the thousands of healthcare executives at the conference, the particular session I was in to learn from the FDA about the SNAP program had less than five participants. When I returned from the conference I couldn't wait to share what I had learned with my team, peers, and my non-profit Board colleagues at our local Loaves and Fishes organization.

While it has been a slow process, our community has been receptive to finding ways to create access to food in addition to access to healthcare. In addition to serving on the team to merge our local pantry system (Loaves and Fishes) with our local Meals on Wheels (Friendship Trays), we also added food pharmacies, mobile pantries, food shares, and at home delivery to our tool kit to help close the gap between the supply of good food and people who need it.

While all of these are valiant, meaningful efforts—and many communities can tout the same—we do not have one reliable system in place which ensures access to quality food for all Americans. Chronic diseases account for 70% of all deaths in America [3]. Poor diet is directly correlated to obesity, heart disease, and type 2 diabetes.

Drawing back to our earlier example, children age out of structured healthcare with wellness and behavioral tools; children age out of meal programs when they graduate high school but may be eligible for programs such as SNAP. What systems do we have in place within public health and healthcare to help this transition from child to adult with intention to provide a stable foundation of health?

Illuminating the Successes of Healthcare and Public Health Together

We need to question the decisions being made and distribution of resources based upon the data and science. Is funding aligned to the policies, programs, and behavior which will truly drive health? Health for all or health for some?

We've all heard the reasons why the current system exists. We all may have our favorites—policy, resources, incentives, access, outcomes, leadership, will, etc. This book will not provide the systemic research on the reasons. This book serves as an illumination of the distinct attributes of each practice, medicine and public health, partnered with business to provide a roadmap for joining the forces of these great practices to unify efforts in a complex and overwhelming system. This book intends to celebrate the differences between healthcare and public health while raising our consideration of their power together. Then we give a simple call to action for us to do it—join hands, join expertise, join data, join systems—to focus on efforts to validate more specifically the drivers of health and its ROI, and to improve outcomes for the individuals and the community.

This book also acknowledges and celebrates those who have demonstrated the promise of this partnership of medicine and public health with measurable ROI being made. We will highlight their work and also ask the mandatory questions of its scalability and sustainability—including the value proposition/business case. Yes, I said it: business case! Many are striking the balance of health, care, and business. I believe most want to; our challenge is to create a system which makes us stop and ask why we ever thought we could or should go it alone.

References:

1) Gunderson GW. *The National School Lunch Program:
    Background and Development*. Nova Publishers; 2003.

2) Courtemanche C, Denteh A, Tchernis R. Estimating the
    associations between SNAP and food insecurity, obesity, and
    food purchases with imperfect administrative measures of
    participation. *Southern Economic Journal*. 2019;86(1):202-228.

3) Raghupathi W, Raghupathi V. An empirical study ofchronic
    approach. International Journal of Environmental Research
    and Public Health. 2018;15(3):431.
    https://doi.org/10.3390/ijerph15030431

What is Public Health?
What is Medicine?

Healthcare and Public Health are Necessarily Intertwined: The Social Determinates of Health

RESEARCH FROM THE Kaiser Family Foundation notes that efforts in the US have traditionally looked to the healthcare system as the key driver of health and health outcomes. However, there is broader understanding and acceptance of other drivers in our health including social, economic, and environmental factors. Although there has been significant progress in recognizing and addressing the range of determinants of health, challenges remain as we have yet to implement sustainable systems to reliably address these drivers. Notably, any efforts require working across siloed sectors with separate funding streams, varied incentives, and access to data and analytics.

The figure below from the Kaiser Foundation is a simple description of the elements included in the determinants of health, including the healthcare system [1]. I find this figure helpful as it is comprehensive but simple. As we embark on understanding, questioning, and purposefully changing the current system, it is extremely beneficial to have a common description and definition of the social determinates of health. This is one of the best I have found so I share with you as a working definition. As we first seek to understand the current state of our systems, it is valuable to level set on the core competencies of both the practice of public health and the practice of medicine—there is so much overlap between these two practices!

Social Determinants of Health

Economic Stability	Neighborhood and Physical Environment	Education	Food	Community and Social Context	Health Care System
Employment	Housing	Literacy	Hunger	Social integration	Health coverage
Income	Transportation	Language	Access to healthy options	Support systems	Provider availability
Expenses	Safety	Early childhood education		Community engagement	Provider linguistic and cultural competency
Debt	Parks				
Medical bills	Playgrounds	Vocational training		Discrimination	
Support	Walkability				Quality of Care
		Higher education			

Health Outcomes
Mortality, Mobility, Life Expectancy, Health Care Expenditures, Health Status, Functional Limitations

Source: Kaiser Family Foundation [1].

Addressing the Social Determinates of Health in Healthcare: An Example

When we focus on the social determinates of health, we begin to illuminate opportunities to improve people's lives. Here is an example of doing just that, through joining the systems of healthcare and public health.

When I was a young executive responsible for the operations of a busy Level 1 Emergency Department (ED), I was approached by two of our female attendings to talk about interpersonal violence and violent crime. The research they shared showed a staggering 30% of patients visiting the emergency department were impacted by interpersonal violence. It may not be the main reason for their visit on that particular day, but the person's life was impacted generally by the circumstances of interpersonal violence. Further discussion with the ED team validated the research subjectively. We talked to the nurses and techs and asked them about their experience interacting with patients and families every day. We also asked them about seeing the indicators of interpersonal violence. They saw signs and symptoms of the disease of interpersonal violence, just as they saw the signs and symptoms of chest pain or upper respiratory infection. Why, then, were we not armed to help address the social determinant of health along with the physical determinant of health? While we explored our options to be part of the solution, the opinions of the staff spanned the spectrum: "We need to have a plan to help every person," "This isn't really our job, especially if it's not related to their medical chief complaint," "I want to help but I don't have time, training, resources ..." You get the point.

From the person/patient's perspective, they live their lives every moment inextricably linked to ALL of the inputs and outputs. The person can't compartmentalize or escape the interconnectedness. The patient may have come to see us because they had chest pain or a UTI, but those symptoms aren't the only things they are bringing with them. The environment they live in, the stressors they experience, and the joy they experience all impact the person, always, regardless of the particular health condition they are experiencing.

Fast forward to our solution: we recognized our patients deserved our help. We knew we could heal or save their lives, but we also were not experts on assisting victims of interpersonal violence and violent crime for the issues unrelated to their physical impact. As is typical, our Emergency Medicine physicians and our entire ED team had an established relationship with the police and sheriff's office. We were already inextricably linked to serve our missions every day, every moment. However, the police department, crime lab, and District Attorney's office could perhaps see more clearly the role we could play in healthcare to help advocate for victims and catch the perpetrators. We built upon these relationships to formalize our conversation with the leadership to discuss the issue, learn more about it together, and decide what could and should be done about it.

I was very young in my career, and I remember receiving the call from the Deputy Chief of Police at the time, welcoming me to join the meeting, and, later, asking me to chair the board as we formalized our partnership, work, and impact together. This included our local police, crime lab, sheriff, district attorney (DA), community college, the competitive hospital system, and the community organization combating interpersonal violence. Together, we learned about what we were each doing and talked about how we could do it better together. We looked at the science, the drivers from the population, and individual perspectives clinical, social, and behavior conditions—and learned about the potential gaps in our system.

Our solution was to establish a 24/7 volunteer program trained by the community interpersonal violence organization, so the healthcare team could have a new tool in their toolkit to "treat" the patient. This consisted of an interpersonal violence expert to come in and help assist the patient with the resources they needed to support their social symptoms. The crime lab and DA office trained the staff—ED and OR—to preserve evidence while they saved lives to further assist the DA prosecute the bad guys. Our local community college introduced courses on forensic medicine training, including photography, so individuals could pursue expertise and students could explore professions in the field.

The cost was minimal. We all pitched in to hire a program coordinator, but each agency already had the expertise. The innovation was this: we realized the missing piece was the integration of our expertise and the availability of tools to address the medical and public health symptoms. We created viable treatment options integrated into the workflow spanning the medical and public health continuum.

We created measurements to ensure our shared goals of helping treat victims, catch and change the community system to align incentives by which we all approached interpersonal violence together. Once this was established, we were proud to be one of the first hospitals in America to introduce universal screening for interpersonal violence at triage. One of our first successes was the conviction of Ray Carruth in the murder of Cherica Adams and near death of his unborn baby. Our DA stated that, if it were not for the evidence preserved by the medical team, a conviction would have been difficult. Powerful.

We did not sit down and talk about how we were going to profit, or how the overall financials were going to work until AFTER we were educated about the current environment and systems. The ROI can be measured in multiple ways. From a straight investment perspective, the new investment was no more than $250K annually, including a program director, social worker, office space, and overhead. From the healthcare systems perspective, the ED recidivism dropped by at least 10% percent, with an estimated net savings of $500K per year. For the police department and DA office, the rapidity of test collection, efficacy of evidence, and increased conviction rate was also a net gain. For the community agency, the education and systemic underpinning of helping those in need was all net margin.

One final note on this example: this program was established in the early 2000s and is still going strong two decades later, serving millions of people.

Unifying for Overall Health

Take another example: women have been having babies forever. Obstetricians have known for decades that a measurable percentage of women will suffer from postpartum depression. However, it was rare even a decade ago to have this addressed during your medical care proactively as a pregnant woman. Similar to the interpersonal violence example above, the medical teams were aware of the incidence of the mental health likelihood, but when queried as to why it was not directly addressed, the lack of time, training, and accountability to responsibility beyond the traditional medical model was apparent. It wasn't that the medical team didn't care or didn't know, but their training and the tools readily available were not made to address the behavioral health component. However, when we were able to provide easier access to a

Additive medicine solutions and additive public health solutions will not necessarily drive the improvements we need.

team and tools trained to address postpartum depression, we enlarged the treatment options to include medical and behavioral health so the patient's health could be addressed holistically. This is an example of matching resources and expertise to address the reality of the situation, and it's driven by the science of the incidence of needs in the population as well as individuals. It can and is being done.

Additive medicine solutions and additive public health solutions will not necessarily drive the improvements we need. Breaking apart our body and the influences in our life has not served us well to date. But it is enormously overwhelming to balance the factors which drive our overall health. This is where our subject matter expertise developed to date and the promise of data/analytics and artificial intelligence can help us take an otherwise fragmented and overwhelming puzzle, apply business and financial principles along with new incentives to thoughtfully question the traditional models, and bring some clarity for focus and action. There are not limitless resources, nor can community and individuals tolerate constant change, especially in deeply engrained traditions and habits. However, we have enough resources invested currently in the systems of public health and medicine to question its effectiveness. It is time to critically consider and make the changes we need to make to improve health for individuals and the communities.

Training and Tools: Public Health

Exploring the history of public health, we see that it is the science of protecting and improving the health of people and their communities. The practice is focused upon promoting healthy lifestyles, researching disease and injury prevention, and detecting, preventing, and responding to infectious disease. While public health is focused on protecting the health of entire populations, the populations can be defined in different ways, for example as small as a neighborhood or as large as a county or country. Public health also recognizes limiting health disparities.

There are about 60 accredited schools of public health and 100 accredited public health programs in the United States [2]. The training underpinning public health degrees includes epidemiology, biostatistics, social and behavior science, environmental health, and health policy and management.

The tools by which the training is applied includes policy development, education, human behavior change, and community advocacy.

The outcomes metrics of public health include increased life expectancy, increased quality of life, and disease prevention.

The Top Ten Great Public Health Achievements—United States, 1900–1999 [3]

- Vaccination
- Motor-vehicle safety
- Safer workplaces
- Control of infectious diseases
- Decline in deaths from coronary heart disease and stroke
- Safer and healthier foods
- Healthier mothers and babies
- Family planning
- Fluoridation of drinking water
- Recognition of tobacco use as a health hazard

Training and Tools: Medicine

The practice of medicine is the science and art dealing with the maintenance of health and the prevention, alleviation, or cure of a disease. The practice is focused upon the individual, diagnosing disease, and aligning treatment to address the diagnosis.

There are about 192 accredited schools of medicine in the United States; 155 MD-granting institutions and 37 DO-granting institutions. The training underpinning medical degrees include anatomy, biochemistry, microbiology, pathology, and pharmacology.

The tools by which the training is applied in medicine includes doctor visits, procedures, and prescriptions.

The outcomes metrics of medicine include quality and safety, patient experience, efficiency, and provider satisfaction.

Top Medical Successes in History [4]

- Vaccines (1796)
- Anesthesia (1846)
- Germ therapy (1861)
- Medical imaging (1895)
- Penicillin (1928)
- Organ transplants (1954)
- Antiviral drugs (1960)
- Stem cell therapy (1970)
- Immunotherapy (1970)
- Artificial intelligence (21st century)

Definitions of Quality: Two Different Perspectives

One final piece I found in my research which was interesting is the definition of quality. I speak to outcomes metrics above, but the validation of quality should be part of this conversation as well. By understanding the public health and healthcare definition of quality, we can further examine their complimentary nature and common ground.

In healthcare, quality is determined by six key aims provided in the Institute of Medicine report Crossing the Quality Chasm: A New Health System for the 21st Century [5]. Meanwhile, aims that characterize public health quality are set forth in a consensus report by the Department of Health and Human Services, Office of Public Health and Science: Consensus Statement on Quality in the Public Health System (2008).

Healthcare	Public Health
• Patient-centered	• Population-centered
• Timely	• Proactive
• Equitable	• Equitable
• Safe	• Health-promoting
• Efficient	• Efficient
• Effective	• Effective
	• Transparent
	• Risk-reducing
	• Vigilant

Source: Quality/Crawley [6]

Public Health and Medicine, Together?

In America, there are over 80 programs which facilitate physicians obtaining dual degrees in medicine and public health. The fundamentals are in place for education on each of the sciences, but when I do research to pull up how public health and medicine tout their advances together, the Google search is grim. The research is a bit more robust, but research to practical application still seems to be a gap that, if filled, may yield tremendous results for our health trajectory as a nation.

I spoke to several physicians who also achieved a PhD in public health or a Masters in Public Health (MPH). Overwhelmingly all were grateful for the scientific understanding of populations to compliment training in medicine focused on individuals. Many also implemented into their practice elements of medicine and public health, largely in the area of prevention, and most commonly in the area of oncology and pediatrics as discussed earlier. Furthermore, many voiced their agreement that the actual practice of both exist in systems which were largely separate—forcing individuals to focus on a medical track or public health track. Not many could bring up examples where they were using both medical and public health science and tools robustly and reliably together. We did uncover some great examples, and we will spend time later in this book diving deeper into the operations and practice of medicine and public health together. This is the whole purpose—to illuminate how medicine and public health can and should be practiced together—raising the potential to achieve positive, sustainable outcomes of health not just for some and not just some of the time, but for all, as much of the time as possible.

Perspectives of Medicine and Public Health

The differences shown in the tables on the next page speak to the underlying ways both fields are training to define and relate to health as a whole. Where healthcare is focused on giving the individual patient medical care when necessary, public health emphasizes prevention and keeping populations healthy to reduce the need for later interventions.

Medicine	Public Health
Primary focus on individual	Primary focus on population
Personal service ethic, conditioned by awareness of social responsibilities	Public service ethic, tempered by concerns for the individual
Emphasis on diagnosis and treatment, care for the whole patient	Emphasis on prevention, health promotion for the whole community
Medical paradigm places predominant emphasis on medical care	Public health paradigm employs a spectrum of interventions aimed at the environment, human behavior and lifestyle, and medical care
Well established profession with sharp public image	Multiple professional identities with diffuse public image
Uniform system for certifying specialists beyond professional medical degree	Variable certification of specialists beyond professional public health degree
Lines of specialization organized, for example, by organ system (cardiology, neurology); patient group (obstetrics, pediatrics); etiology and pathophysiology (infectious diseases, oncology); technical skill (radiology, surgery)	Lines of specialization organized, for example, by analytic method (epidemiology, toxicology); setting and population (occupational health, international health); substantive health problem (environmental health, nutrition)
Biological sciences central, stimulated by needs of patients, move between laboratory and bedside	Biological sciences central, stimulated by major threats to health of populations; move between laboratory and field

Source: American Journal of Preventive Medicine [7]

On the one hand, the healthcare system is largely focused on sick care. There are of course exceptions, including early childhood medical protocols, screening for cancer such as mammograms and colonoscopies, and increasing interest and pressure to head towards overall health. And equity. However, the incentives of healthcare lend towards sick care. On the other hand, the incentives of public health lend towards underserved populations. Both are not enough and both innately create a gap in how health is considered as a whole [8].

Physician Leaders are Essential

Physicians interact with individuals and families every day, giving them a real-world perspective of how people live. Therefore, our physicians are in a unique position to help us recast the way we approach health from the lens of the individual.

Let's follow the power in the current system. If 80% of health funds are spent on healthcare, where does the power and influence sit in healthcare? While administrative overhead and leadership positions account for 20% of the healthcare overhead, anyone in healthcare realizes that change in healthcare is driven largely by physicians [9]. This is especially true if the changes we are trying to champion have to do with the tools available to "prescribe" new solutions that will help people address their holistic health. This means not just their care or sick care, but to expand our tool kit to include solutions that will address the social, physical, and behavioral determinants of health. In total. The buy-in and leadership of the physician is critical to augment the care pathway and position the physician to endorse a "treatment" to the individual which may not be the traditional medical treatment but rather a social or behavioral treatment.

Public Health Leaders are Essential

In public health, the understanding of the population from the macro perspective has to be matched with real world input from those in the community for the interventions to be effective. The process of public health practice typically involves the leadership of the community to validate the needs and in turn the intervention. Community stakeholders provide validity on the appropriateness and feasibility of the intervention. Additionally, their insight and guidance are critical in not only accessing the target population but gaining the trust of the community and providing feedback and ongoing recommendations.

Bringing this Leadership Together

Both professions are rooted in their service to improve health, but the often disparate ways the interventions are studied, validated, applied, and measured is cause not only for concern but also for questions. Communities are made up of individuals and individuals makeup a community. Both are inextricably linked, but we often act as if they are separate.

The fundamental understanding of the training and tools of both professions is essential as we start to build the case for their power together. There are too many opportunities for people to "talk" or present themselves as subject matter experts. If you pull back the curtain, however, there is not the training nor the efficacy of reliable systems to drive the outcomes we need and deserve. A physician would question a public health professional discussing treatment and medical procedures if they are not a practicing physician caring for patients; in turn, public health professionals would question physicians who talk about population characteristics and disease progression at a population level if they did not have real world experience studying the population, trends, and comparative analytics.

In summary, below is a culmination of our research and learnings in an easy to reference table noting the training, tools, and outcomes metrics of both Medicine and Public Health.

	Medicine	Public Health
Outcome Metrics (current)	Disease Management/Cure Morbidity Mortality	Reduce Exposure/Risk Factors Disease Incidence Mortality
Tools	Doctor's Visit Hospital/ED Visits Procedures Pharmacology Case/Care Management	Policy Behavior Change Clean Water/Air Violence Intervention Community Health Worker
Training	Anatomy Physiology Pharmacology	Epidemiology Biostatistics Human Behavior

Kaney 2022

There is nothing necessarily wrong with continuing as we are—each with a casual glance towards each other when things like a pandemic pop up. Or obtaining joint training in both fields but entering systems which fragment the practice, including competing incentives, funding, leadership, and advocacy. To date, the traditional systems of healthcare and public health largely ignore what is not their subject matter expertise. The reason for this book is to help illuminate what a problem this is—and, with the willpower to join forces moving forward, we can integrate best practice programs aimed to positively impact the factors and accelerate the outcomes without additional funding. In fact, the premise is the expenditure would be less because the interventions would more accurately address the factors driving health.

Seize the Moment

Let's ask ourselves where there are reliable systems in which medical and public health scientists coexist as common practice with shared data, incentives, goals, and platforms to deliver solutions to individuals and populations. There are plenty of organizations and people in the medical and public health arena trying to bridge the expertise and help provide reliable solutions for individuals and populations. However, the systems of public health and medicine are not built to capitalize on their synergies. It is more a divide and conquer relationship with a clear division of power, instead of a joining of sciences to create a seamless view into the data, trends, and ultimate solutions.

I had a conversation with a former boss who is the Chief Clinical Officer of a large healthcare system in the South. During the pandemic, he was tapped to be the incident commander to lead systems response. While talking about our thoughts on public health and medicine together, he recounted to me one of the very first meetings he attended in March 2020 as the pandemic was quickly becoming a reality. Included in the meeting was the Director of Public Health for his county. They related a robust plan on paper about contact tracing and data collection to support the community efforts. While the plan looked good on paper, it was soon apparent that local public health organizations, while well intended, did not have the resources or expertise to implement such a program. Furthermore, my former boss reflected on perhaps the most important lesson learned that day: it was the first time most in the room—including the Chief Clinical Officer and Public Health Director—had ever met.

But what an opportunity we have to seize the moment. Again, back to the data—the outcomes in America are not what they should be. If leaders across industries are willing to take a critical look at their subject matter expertise and how it can be amplified by integrating with complimentary practices, we should have a shot at changing the trajectory of overall health in America, in addition to spending less money by avoiding duplication, illuminating not only interventions but their measurable impact, or lack thereof, and continuously learning through the data/analytics to refine where our resources will yield the most good. It will take focus, a willingness to question the norm, a relentless eye to cause/effect of policy and funding, and accountability in the whole for what each profession is contributing to the health of America. This is a time for real change, systemic change—not just incremental change. People and communities deserve it and they are counting on us.

References:

1) Artiga S, Hinton E. Beyond health care: The role of social
    determinants in promoting health and health equity. KFF.org.
    Published May 10, 2018. Accessed February 4, 2022.
    https://www.kff.org/racial-equity-and-health-policy/issue-
    brief/beyond-health-care-the-role-of-social-determinants-
    in-promoting-health-and-health-equity/.

2) List of accredited schools and programs. CEPH.org.
    Accessed March 10, 2022. https://ceph.org/about/org-
    info/who-we-accredit/accredited/.

3) Ten great public health achievements—United States, 1900-
    1999. CDC.gov. Published April 2, 1999. Accessed January 15,
    2022. https://www.cdc.gov/mmwr/preview/mmwrhtml/
    00056796.htm.

4) Top ten medical advances in history. Proclinical.com.
    Published June 21, 2021. Accessed January 15, 2022.
    https://www.proclinical.com/blogs/2021-6/the-top-10-
    medical-advances-in-history.

5) Institute of Medicine (US) Committee on Quality of Health
    Care in America. *Crossing the Quality Chasm: A New Health
    System for the 21st Century.* National Academies Press
    (US);2001.

6) Cowley C. What quality improvement means to healthcare
    and public Health. NICHQ.org. Accessed January 22, 2022.
    https://www.nichq.org/insight/what-quality-improvement-
    means-healthcare-and-public-health.

7) Maeshiro R, Koo D, Keck CW. Integration of public health into medical education: an introduction to the supplement. *Am J Prev Med.* 2011;41:S306-S308.

8) Schneider EC, Shah A, Doty MM, Tikkanen R, Fields K, Williams II RD. Mirror mirror 2021 reflecting poorly: Healthcare in the U.S. compared to other high-income countries. The Commonwealth Fund; August 2021. Accessed January 15, 2022. https://collections.nlm.nih.gov/catalog/nlm:nlmuid-9918300978506676-pdf.

9) Porter ME, Lee TH. The strategy that will fix healthcare. *Harvard Business Review.* Published October 2013. Accessed January 22, 2022. https://hbr.org/2013/10/the-strategy-that-will-fix-health-care.

What is Health?

Multiple Definitions of Health

THE DEFINITION OF health in the research is important to understand. If our goal is to improve health, we need to be unified in what health is, how it's measured, and what drives it.

Not to oversimplify, but perhaps our lack of alignment on the definition of health is the root of the problem. We are all playing a different sport with a different scoreboard. Or we are all part of an orchestra but playing off different scores.

Everyone in America understands the definition of poverty objectively in a dollar figure. Differing state by state, region by region, poverty is comparing a person or family's income to a threshold or minimum amount of income needed to cover basic needs. But simply put, poverty is lacking the resources to provide the necessities of life—food, clean water, shelter, and clothing. It's much more than just percentage of income. There is data which defines such and the very systems by which state and federal funding is distributed is related directly back to the definition.

For health, is there a shared, agreed upon definition? We noted in the first chapter Kaiser's summary of the determinants of health as a starting point. Let's dive a little deeper.

Public health has a definition and set of measures encompassed in the Community Health Needs Assessment and ranked by state and county boards to note health performance. Healthcare is a bit more complicated. There are subsets of regulatory bodies which measure health outcomes and these outcomes are more developed for hospitals/post-acute sites than for ambulatory settings. As more newly developed care models using nonclinical teammates or community resources, and modes of care such as hospital-at-home and virtual emerge as scalable and viable tools to reach patients and communities, health outcomes specific to these models will need to be developed. The federal and state government are fundamental components to the alignment of health, its definition, measurement, drivers, tools, and incentives to drive improved outcomes. More on this later.

PUBLIC HEALTH Definition of HEALTH

What is health according to public health? Directly from the Centers of Disease Control "The science and art of preventing disease, prolonging life and promoting health through the organized efforts and informed choices of society, organizations, public and private communities and individuals." [1]

MEDICAL/HEALTHCARE Definition of HEALTH

What is the medical definition of health? "Health is a state of complete physical, mental and social well-being and not merely the absence of disease or infirmity." [2]

COMMUNITY Definition of HEALTH

What is the community definition of health? The environmental, social and economic resources to sustain emotional and physical well-being among people in ways that advance their aspirations and satisfy their needs in their unique environments [2].

INDIVIDUAL Definition of HEALTH

What is the individual definition of health? Humans define health as "a state of balance, an equilibrium that an individual has established within himself and between himself and his social and physical environment." [2]

There are various opinions about what is health and, furthermore, what is controllable by populations and individuals. In my opinion, that is fair and it is okay, however, if our goal is drive health for populations and individuals, it is instead necessary to agree upon and align to the factors which drive health so we can help determine which efforts will yield the best results. This may very well be different with a population lens versus an individual lens. Again, that is okay—in fact, that is to be expected. Our hope is that, by validating both perspectives, we can find common ground to join interventions for the greater good of people and populations.

The Factors Affecting Health Outcomes

While there is widespread understanding that the health system and other factors—social determinants—affect health, we know relatively little about their precise contributions to health differences across a population at a point in time or differences in health of a fixed population over time. A literature review by Frakt (2019) looks at research from as far back as the 1970s and provides a historical background to quantify the contribution of various factors of health, which are summarized below. The included studies organize the factors that affect health into five categories: behaviors, medical care, social circumstances, environment, and genetics (the last three are grouped together in the chart, for convenience).

Range of Empirical Estimates for Factors That Affect Health

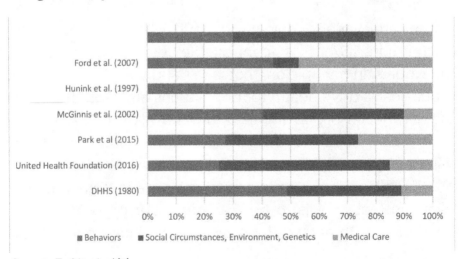

Source: Frakts et. al. [3]

Frakt's literature review showcases that neither the focuses of health care nor the focuses of public health alone ever comprise more than 50% of total health. At the start of this book, we referenced the Kaiser Foundation and their research of clinical care driving less than 10% of outcomes but consuming over 80% of the expenditure [4]. The bottom line is simple: we have to look at both public health and medicine to effectively serve health outcomes. There is no perfect answer or agreement on the weight of impact and it is okay. I would advise us to not spend so much time debating the percentages. What is most important is realizing that there are several factors which drive health, and all are interconnected. We have known this for decades, and it has not only been validated but now talked about at a more frequent occurrence. Furthermore, utilizing the research to estimate a framework by which we weight the factors is intended to help drive purposeful intervention, not perfection.

Combining our understanding of health outcomes and factors, the summary below from the Country Rankings created by the University of Wisconsin Population Health Institute [5] helps to frame how we can use the knowledge of the outcomes and drivers of health in the broad framework to overlay the practice of medicine and public health. With that said, this summary is a little light, in my opinion, on health outcomes. The already referenced framework from Kaiser Family Foundation [6] provides more detail about health outcomes; however, the expenditures in this framework should take into account all health expenditures, not just healthcare expenditures.

County Health Rankings

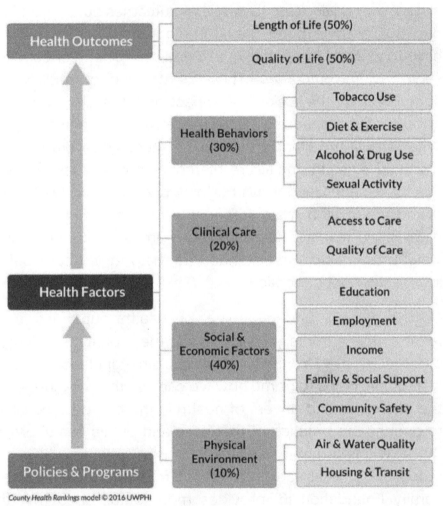

County Health Rankings model © 2016 UWPHI

Source: The University of Wisconsin Population Health Institute. County Health Rankings & Roadmaps, 2022.

Kaiser Family Foundation: Driving Factors of Health and Longevity

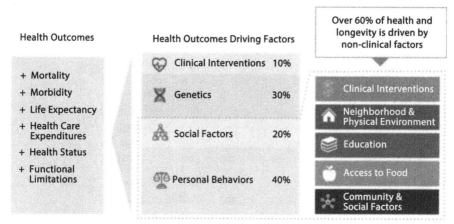

Source: _Kaiser Family Foundation_, Beyond Health Care: The Role of Social Determinants in Promoting Health and Health Equity, 5/18

Healthcare Spending in the US

When compared to the rest of the world, the US is often criticized for spending twice as much on health with mediocre outcomes. Much research has been done in this arena as well, and the apples-to-apples comparison is often difficult since countries approach health and healthcare differently, categorizing healthcare and social services differently. In countries with socialized medicine, the funding and approach is more integrated into the social services fabric and vice versa. I thought it helpful to provide a high level overview of the spending to help us further educate ourselves and provide insight into where the power of spending lies now. This will allow us to question if the spending aligns with what we know as the factors in total driving health.

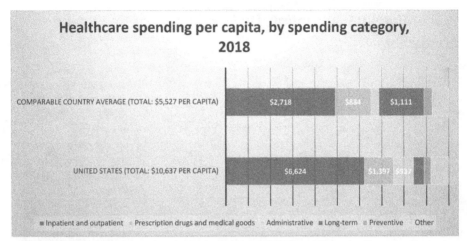

Healthcare spending per capita, by spending category, 2018

Note: Comparable countries include Austria, Belgium. Canada, France, Germany, Netherlands, Sweden, Switzerland, and the United Kingdom

Source: KFF analysis of OEDC Health Statistics; Peterson KFF Health System Tracker[7]

The funding for health is skewed towards health care and less money is spent on prevention.

Healthcare economics and incentives are complicated. In re-reading Fuchs "Who Shall Live" originally written in the early 1970s [8], the problems of healthcare have been around for decades. In a fee for service system or margin driven organization, resources, while plenty for some, are not limitless. Decisions have to be made about how to invest and maintain margin and outcomes. Healthcare decision making over the last several decades has created a system where resources, access, trust, and alignment are maldistributed. Urban vs rural; rich vs poor; white vs black/brown. Almost any measuring stick will demonstrate gaps in both public health and healthcare services. Furthermore, funds for public health have diminished over time, as has the role of public health leadership in the overall call to action on the drivers of health, not just healthcare, within each community. However, the hope is by aligning a population health view with a healthcare view, we can focus in on the key drivers and tailor solutions aligned with the incentives in the financial system to change prioritization and tools used to address the issues at hand.

The pandemic has skewed the traditional fund and spend trajectory. Most of the recent health spending growth is in insurance programs, both private and public. Private insurance expenditures now represent 27.9% of total health spending (up from 20.4% in 1970), and public insurance (which includes Medicare, Medicaid, CHIP, and the Veterans Administration and Department of Defense) represented 40.2% of overall health spending in 2020 (up from 22% in 1970). Although out-of-pocket costs per capita have generally been rising, compared to previous decades, they now make up a smaller share of total health expenditures [9].

Total national health expenditures grew by nearly $365 billion in 2020 compared to 2019. About one-third (nearly $119 billion) of that growth in spending can be attributed to the increase in spending on public health, which includes federal spending to develop COVID-19 vaccines under Operation Warp Speed, strategic stockpiles of drugs and vaccines, and health facility preparedness. An increase in hospital expenditures contributed 20.9% of the growth, which reflects increased federal payments and loans to hospitals for COVID-19 relief (through the Provider Relief Fund and Paycheck Protection Program), as well as increased Medicaid spending. Meanwhile, health spending on dental services and research, structures, and equipment declined from the prior year [9].

Spending on public health activities and federal programs including the Provider Relief Fund and Paycheck Protection Program drove the 9.7% increase in overall health spending from 2019 to 2020; when these spending categories are excluded, overall health spending increased only 1.9% from 2019 to 2020. Health services spending plunged early in the pandemic as care was delayed or cancelled [9].

Perhaps some of the recent shifts in funding and spending, including the creation of new relationships across medicine and public health, can serve as a launching pad for creating a new system of health together.

Addressing these Factors in Practice

Speaking with hundreds of public health and medical professionals, there is an understanding of what each does—kind of. There is also an increased acknowledgement and growing understanding there are several factors which drive health.

Medical people reference their community health training and the word prevention is commonplace. Public health professionals will reference prevention as well, specifically primary care, and note children's care as a gold standard with immunizations and standing protocols for comprehensive health assessments for newborn to roughly age eighteen. What you don't hear as much about, from either community, is how these communities intersect—or could intersect—or need to intersect more to build upon the current success and be even more effective. The economic alignment is not clear, the value is not crystalized, and the incentives to pursue are not readily seen.

But the similarities help define some of the intersections between these two, and there is a movement to align them more closely. Both groups acknowledge the need for equity, efficiency, and efficacy. Moreover, healthcare has a burgeoning focus on preventive interventions and the social determinants of health. While those aren't yet widespread approaches, they indicate a desire for healthcare to evolve how it addresses patient issues. The point is and will be

We should, however, challenge our application of our science and current solutions against the broader framework of health.

through this book, we are not starting from scratch on any of this and we should not. We should, however, challenge our application of our science and current solutions against the broader framework of health.

References:

1) What is public health? CDCfoundation.org. Accessed January 31, 2022. https://www.cdcfoundation.org/what-public-health.

2) Satorius N. The meanings of health and its promotion. *Croat Med J.* 2006;47(4):662-664. https://www.ncbi.nlm.nih.gov/pmc/articles/PMC2080455/

3) Frakt A, Jha A, Glied S, Raphael K. What is known about the drivers of health: A literature review. Harvard Global Health Institute. Accessed January 31, 2022. https://driversofhealth.org/wp-content/uploads/SDH.whitepaper_v8.pdf.

4) What makes us healthy vs what we spend on being healthy. Bipartisanpolicy.org. Published June 5, 2012. Accessed January 31, 2022. https://bipartisanpolicy.org/report/what-makes-us-healthy-vs-what-we-spend-on-being-healthy/.

5) 2022 County health ranking national findings report. Countyhealthrankings.org. Accessed January 13, 2022. https://www.countyhealthrankings.org/reports/2022-county-health-rankings-national-findings-report.

6) Artiga S, Hinton E. Beyond health care: The role of social determinants in promoting health and health equity. KFF.org. Published May 10, 2018. Accessed February 4, 2022. https://www.kff.org/racial-equity-and-health-policy/issue-brief/beyond-health-care-the-role-of-social-determinants-in-promoting-health-and-health-equity/.

7) Kurani N and Cox C. What drives health spending in the U.S. compared to other countries? HealthSystemTracker.org. Published September 25, 2020. Accessed March 21, 2022. https://www.healthsystemtracker.org/brief/what-drives-health-spending-in-the-u-s-compared-to-other-countries/.

8) Fuchs VR. *Who Shall Live? Health Economic and Social Choice*. World Scientific;2011.

9) Kurani N, Ortaliza J, Wager E, Fox L, Amin K. How has U.S. spending on healthcare changed over time? Published February 25, 2022. Accessed November 29, 2022. https://www.healthsystemtracker.org/chartcollection/u-s-spending-healthcare-changed-time.

How Are We Doing So Far?

Equity as a Measure of Success

A PREFACE FOR this section is needed to describe me and my leadership style. I am affectionately referred to as a hard grader. As I have done my research for this book, I am glad I am a hard grader. Serving in professions such as public health and healthcare, it is our calling to help those who are counting on us. While there are pockets of excellence, we have not arrived. I am also not convinced we are aligned on the systemic changes needed to really drive a difference, more positive, equitable outcome. So—how are we doing?

Noting all of the contributions, training, successes and attributes we have within our systems—our outcomes are mediocre at best. Reflecting back on the Kaiser Family Foundation, let's look at a snapshot of America's trended performance for the Health Outcomes Measures.

Health Outcome Metric	2000	2010	2018	+/-
Death Rate per 100K	869.0	747.0	723.6	-145.4
Life Expectancy	76.8	78.7	78.7	+1.9
Healthcare Expenditure (constant 2020 dollars)	$1.945B	$3.008B	$3.701B	+$1.756B
Healthcare Expenditure % of GDP	13.3%	17.2%	17.6%	+4.3%

Source(s): Bastian B, Tejada Vera B, Arias E, et al. Mortality trends in the United States, 1900–2018. National Center for Health Statistics. 2020 [1], Peterson—KFF Health System Tracker [2]

This data is reflective of the average performance, all in. Which means the devil is in the details and it should be. Drop into the details of any one of the metrics, and segment again by urban/rural, white/ black/ brown, income level, gender ... the deviation from the mean performance is startling at best, unacceptable when we truly view the data for what it is showing us. I am a proud member of our profession—both public health and healthcare administration. While I am proud and grateful for some of the work I have been part of and will tout its benefits and lives saved, I am humble enough to know that is not enough. We have not arrived. We are not performing to a reliable standard of excellence we can and should be attaining. Certainly for some, but not for all, and those in poverty or struggling with upward mobility, our work is not providing stable ground by which those who want to can achieve the health they deserve.

I also know running the same set of plays for public health and medicine is not going to achieve a different outcome. It is critical for us to examine the science, let the data tell us the story—the good and the bad—and we must join forces with complimentary disciplines to address reliably all the factors of health.

Creating Equity

In this moment, post pandemic, if healthcare tries to solve the equity issue it created using only healthcare tools alone, it will fail. If public health doesn't enable, implement, and use the scale of their tools, other options will not be believed nor advocated for. If healthcare and public health don't join forces, we will duplicate and water down the science that we already have at our fingertips. Key drivers of the life expectancy surge in the 20th century were better hygiene, development of vaccines and antibiotics, and better diagnosis and treatment of individual diseases. While some of the drivers remain (vaccines), the focus over time has shifted, and it will have to continue to shift. Antibotics used too frequently actually increases disease; overuse of prescription medication can cause healthcare created epidemics like the opioid crisis. Mismanagement of water supplies or environmental safety measures result in people dying or impacted by disease and/ or disaster as we saw in Flint, Michigan and New Orleans during Hurricane Katrina. Rather than focusing on the disease alone, or the community alone, the focus now is around the underlying intersection and interdependence of both. Peter Block's book, *Community: The Structure of Belonging,* [3] was recommended reading for a leadership class focused on driving positive community change. Block discusses the need to work through both—individuals and community—to achieve sustainable results. After all, communities are made up of individuals, and individuals make up communities. Simple—but true. As much as you try to extract the two from each other, it doesn't happen.

The pandemic impacted us all and stayed true to what we have lots of research to support—illness and disease impact Black and Latino people more than White people [4]. It impacts the poor at a higher rate than the rich. Healthcare impacts your overall health by, at the most, 20%. The zip code we live in can come closer to predicting health outcomes often better than metabolic indicators. This narrative is the language of public health. Key lessons learned and the silver lining prioritized by health equity as a strategy for success, utilization of population-based forecasting models, expeditious implementation of a new immunization, large scale distribution of vaccine—the list continues. The PowerPoints are being drafted. The strategic plans will reflect the new normal. The new buzz words are in flight.

But none of this is new. The pandemic simply shined a light on what we already know, and we have known for years. This simply is the opportunity to intentionally align the practice of medicine and the practice of public health. One practice originates from the treatment of the health of the individual and one practice originates from the maintenance of the health of the population, but both practices have similar goals.

Walking the Talk

Healthcare systems are increasingly called to action to address the diversity/inclusion gaps in their programs and workforce, and in also the equity by which they apply their programs and services in the community. This is positive in many ways, but it is also problematic when you consider the tools and expertise healthcare typically has on its bench. They are not necessarily tools of global access and effectiveness from a person/ patient/community point of view. The traditional healthcare system is built with the lens of sick care, and largely to accommodate the practice of physicians, not the viewpoint of the consumer. This statement will make healthcare people bristle, or point to various programs and PowerPoints which highlight programs and changes. But fundamentally, the traditional system of healthcare has not been addressed or the incentives adjusted. Therefore, while many healthcare executives believe in equity, access, and the role they play in creating a better health system, the ways by which a margin is generated and the traditional tools to serve the individuals and community remain largely the same.

Perhaps systems such as Kaiser or states such as Massachusetts who have shifted to more risk-based models with more longitudinal accountability for outcomes and payment can get there. Medicaid and Medicare are trying but progress is slow. Even the VA—which shares many attributes to align incentives and make a go at it—struggles to balance alignment of funding to drive health and provide healthcare. We will highlight in our ending chapters programs and systemic changes which are helping to lead the way in a more holistic approach to health. The work being done in mental health in certain parts of our country give us reason to be optimistic and to emulate the progress the leaders are making.

Public health is having their moment thanks to the pandemic. After years of playing a supporting role and weathering cuts in funding, there is renewed attention and interest in public health. We need to think about how to harness this attention effectively. Public health has excelled in research, academics, and unwavering advocates for equity. Its track record in practice and scalable application beyond vaccines and water and food safety are not as measurable. From a leadership standpoint, while there are many dual trained physicians in medical and public health and more coming by the moment, the ability for a physician who has chosen the public health track to truly influence the care pathway and "treatments" offered to populations and individuals is weak. The public health department leaders are not always as integrated into the overall health equation or, even more importantly, driving the total health conversation from their populations. Many refer to challenges in data, labor, and overall bureaucratic or antiquated systems. However, this can be addressed, especially the access to data and measurements, if there is the political will and focus to do so.

Illuminating the Partnership

As we noted earlier, both public health and medicine claim vaccines as a top success. Vaccination has resulted in the eradication of smallpox; the elimination of poliomyelitis in the Americas; and the control of measles, rubella, tetanus, diphtheria, Haemophilus influenzae type b, and other infectious diseases in the United States and other parts of the world. Most recently with the COVID pandemic, the impact of vaccination—or a pill to prevent severe illness/death—is at the forefront. Washing our hands, wearing a mask, and keeping our distance was almost

> **... both public health and medicine claim vaccines as a top success.**

too simplistic, affordable, and inconvenient for us to get our heads around it as a viable solution. However, all of the interventions are needed—and their importance varied depending on the course of the virus on each population and on each individual. It illuminates the partnership of public health and medicine, one we can use as the catalyst.

Perhaps this is good timing as the pandemic and vaccination have already spurred the conversation of the benefit of public health and medicine, together.

References:

1) Bastian B, Tejada Vera B, Arias E, et al. Mortality trends in the United States, 1900–2018. National Center for Health Statistics. 2020.

2) Kurani N, Ortaliza J, Wager E, Fox L, Amin K. How has U.S. spending on healthcare changed over time? Published February 25, 2022. Accessed November 29, 2022. https://www.healthsystemtracker.org/chartcollection/u-s-spending-healthcare-changed-time.

3) Block P. *Community: The Structure of Belonging.* Berrett-Koehler Publishers;2018.

4) Betancourt JR. Communities of color devastated by COVID-19: Shifting the narrative. Harvard Health Blog. Published October 22, 2020. Accessed April 2, 2022. https://www.health.harvard.edu/blog/communities-of-color-devastated-by-covid-19-shifting-the-narrative-2020102221201.

Better Together?

The Goal of this Moment

LET'S SEE WHERE we stand. We are now educated on the fundamentals of the sciences of public health and medicine, examples of the most successful interventions of each, and we have a working definition of health, including its factors and overarching outcome metrics. This creates a scoreboard of sorts, allowing us to consider the system of health—not just healthcare and not just public health. We now enter the journey of realizing the value of its alignment together.

The goal of this moment is not to start over (have I said that already?). It is to evolve from the current state, using the best practices of each domain so we can create followership and momentum as we join hands of public health and medicine.

Key Components for Moving Forward

Regulations are a key component of prioritization and focus. What is required to be done gets done in big bureaucratic industries, and millions are spent by regulatory agencies to ensure the rules are followed. Organizations such as CMS, The Joint Commission, Federal and State HHS, Public Health regulatory agency will be essential in this process of evolution.

Policy experts work on the fabric by which the federal, state, and local governance is structured. This fabric is critical. But a policy doesn't do the work. It frames the work for other critical parts of the system including government agencies, healthcare systems, managed care, medical groups, non-profits, and community health organizations. All of these players are critical to our progress.

The education system is also critical. Academic institutions train the public health and medical students. What are they learning? How are they trained to understand the definition and drivers of health? The way the scientific practice is taught and applied through the complex system is where the value—both business and personal—should come to life. Once the science frames the evidenced-based "treatment," the subject matter experts need to execute their part, but the SYSTEM needs to incentivize the coordination and integration. Too many in public health and medicine have their own special focus—a hunger fighter, environmental activist, a cardiologist, an internist, a surgeon . . . We do not want to dismiss the need for the specialized expertise, but the specialized expertise often misses the forest for the trees since it largely ignores what is happening out of the wheelhouse. Again—a community can't disengage itself from itself, just as a person can't separate their heart from their brain or their bones from their muscles. It's interconnected, and the SYSTEM must treat health as such, especially as it trains our people.

Funding and money are also critical pieces for us to think about. The flow of money and the funding is in essence the power and change agent of the overall system. I did not start with this because my premise is money is not the barrier: we have plenty of money to solve the issues in front of us. It is the distribution of money and measurement of its impact that is the barrier. So, we must first seek to understand the practice of medicine and public health, its science, tools and outcomes metrics, and then understand the framework of health. Then we can understand how to finance solutions and track our return on investment (ROI).

Which brings me to another critical component: science, supported by data and analytics. There are mounds of data by which we can frame our priorities. How is this data being used? As discussed earlier, what is the definition of health and how are we measuring it? How are we using the data we have to prioritize and act upon the opportunities identified? Data is not the answer but it is an enabler, accelerator, and unifier when used correctly. It creates a playing field where we can all know the game, the rules, and how to win. Or if we are all part of an orchestra, we are actually reading from the same sheets of music, understanding our parts and how we compliment each other.

Furthermore, artificial intelligence provides the ability to distill hundreds of thousands of data points—community health needs assessments, claims, and medical records—to find patterns that can help identify the key drivers of health by individual and population, so solutions from both a medicine and public health lens can be effectively debated, evaluated, and applied.

Population Health Analytics needs to become the common language we use to address health—bringing together medicine and public health.

Overcoming the Inertia of Tradition

Perhaps our largest contributor to our current state is the inertia of tradition. The support of the status quo or incremental changes plagues healthcare and public health. We fight to keep the status quo as if the outcomes we have justify our death grip on the current systems. This has always perplexed me in my work to drive change in healthcare and public health programs. (here comes the hard grader

> **We fight to keep the status quo as if the outcomes we have justify our death grip on the current systems.**

again). We act as if what we have today is the best practice and everything else has to be justified to perfection before change is embraced.

The best example I have of this in my career is the use of telemedicine or virtual care. During my time as an executive with a large integrated delivery network, my team and I were charged with "system care coordination." In essence, helping our large but well-meaning system act as one. We worked hand-in-hand with our physicians and clinicians reviewing the science and the traditional systems by which we cared for people in need of our help. What is working? What wasn't? How could we be more effective? More efficient? This led to the use of technology, exploration of care teams, application of evidenced-based care pathways, and, specifically, diversified means of access in the form of telemedicine.

Foundationally, we approached telemedicine and virtual care with one simple statement—Care is Care. Whether provided in person or by digital means (phone, text, email, video), the standard and quality should not be compromised. That said, if done correctly, the distribution of precious clinical resources should be appropriately applied, driving more proactive and less expensive care. This was also my dissertation topic for my DrPH program at UNC Chapel Hill Gillings School of Global Public Health: "How to Accelerate Physicians Use of Virtual Care." Too bad my implementation strategy did not include a global pandemic as the accelerant!

Having the opportunity to pioneer virtual programs focused on care management, behavioral health, direct-to-consumer primary care, genetics, cardiology, and infectious disease, our approach was that every discipline in medicine could find a safe and meaningful application of virtual across the continuum, preserving quality to diversify the tools we had in our tool kit to serve the patients and communities counting on us. We did it—some disciplines were more willing than others—but over the course of five or so years we emerged with integration into the workflow of all services lines and care areas use of virtual to serve our population.

Interestingly, in the build of our direct-to-consumer (DTC) product, we found at the time that we had more rigor and data around the diagnoses we were treating virtually than we did around the ones we were treating in our office settings. For example, the antibiotic prescription rates were readily available for each virtual diagnosis and all of our virtual providers. This was around 2015, and the rise of independent DTC companies was catching steam. We participated in a conference to discuss our experience with telemedicine, especially setting up a DTC within a healthcare system. We felt it critical to address the quality aspects, including metrics such as technology reliability, further intervention/follow-up needed, antibiotic rates, etc. We were ready to share our data to help drive the conversation of transparency, and most importantly, the idea that new advances can be BETTER and MORE effective than the status quo. The for-profits were not willing to share their data so they dropped out. I presented our data to an interesting audience— a majority questioning the efficacy of the new model, the minority touting its value. In retrospect, the additional panel member should have been the tool of the doctor's office visit so we could compare the traditional to the new care model— not peg the new against the new. In my system, I was comparing the traditional to the new—trying to drive fundamental changes in how we provided care with virtual as a core component: a need-to-have, not a nice-to-have. Hard grader, I give myself a C+ on our work overall because not everyone got to the desired state of face-to-face care and virtual care could be reliably provided and applied based upon safety, efficiency, and consumer preference. But to celebrate the wins ... Cardiology embraced telemedicine and systemically included it in their workflow, physician and clinical contracts, and infrastructure. So did infectious disease, pediatrics, and behavioral health. To this day, I will celebrate each of the physician leaders, executives, and their teams for embracing change and seeing a better way to serve.

Keeping the Forward Movement Going

The pandemic provided the springboard for virtual care/ telemedicine to flourish. Parity was granted, technology platforms were forced to scale and integrate into workflow, and clinical leaders embraced it as a viable means to reach patients if the traditional model is not available. The question of maldistribution of clinical resources and access could now have answers using this means of quality care.

From a public health perspective, the variations in coverage and reliability of WiFi impacted the ability of healthcare to serve. The leaders in education were wrestling with the same issue. No WiFi access for students trying to maintain education online. Did we join forces to help solve the systemic problem together of internet access, or did we go it alone? Education is one of the key social determinants of health. Could we have unified our efforts to help increase WiFi access to support education while at the same time creating new connection points for families who were not tied into the existing healthcare system? Could this have been a way to gain trust, understanding, and open communication? Think about when you manage a colleague up for an open position or provide a letter of reference. Almost the entire referral process in healthcare is a shining example of recommending someone you trust. By extending this respect, you are supporting the colleague, the patient, and the family. Think about the power of creating a sustainable referral system between medicine and public health.

For a new model of care to become standard operations, the respected scientists from both medicine and public health are going to have to advocate for the change. Following the scenario above for the referral process, acceleration of adoption will occur if a physician or trusted professional recommends virtual care to patients. This will support the patients, as well as support each other professionally—a win-win. For the past decade,

> **For a new model of care to become standard operations, the respected scientists from both medicine and public health are going to have to advocate for the change.**

the change management for telemedicine was really focused on providers, not consumers. Across specialties, other than psychiatry, there is not a trend of providing care face-to-face and virtually at a more balanced percentage as part of the clinical practice. This means the change management to change the distribution channels of medicine has not born much fruit, yet.

However, the pandemic provided many more consumers access to the power and promise of telemedicine. Referencing the research from McKinsey, consumer likelihood is not over 60%, while physician likelihood is not yet 40% [1].

Substantial variation exists in share of telehealth claims across specialities.

Share of telehealth of outpatient and office visit claims by specialty (February 2021'), %

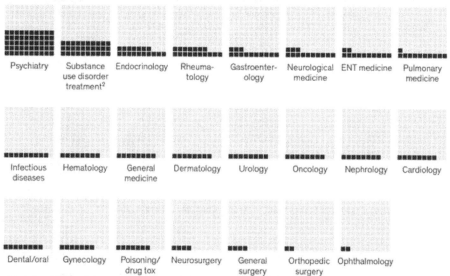

1) Includes only evaluation and management claims; excludes emergency department, hospital inpatient, and physiatry and inpatient claims; excludes certain low-volume specialties.
2) Also includes addiction medicine and addiction treatment.
Source: Compile database; "Telehealth: A quarter-trillion-dollar post-COVID reality?" May 2020, McKinsey.com
Mckinsey analysis

McKinsey
    & Company

The next graph from McKinsey shows the disparity between consumer adoption and physician adoption. The pandemic provided many more consumers access to the power and promise of telemedicine—consumer likelihood is over 60%; while physician likelihood is not yet 40%. This means the individual and population are restless, so perhaps the consumer demand for more choices for medical distribution will be the driving factor of change.

Beliefs about telehealth, % of respondents in agreement with statement

	Convenience	Experience	Usage	Entry point
Patients	60	55	40	63

chose telehealth because it was more convenient	are much more satisfied with telehealth care vs in-person care	will continue to use telehealth after pandemic	are interested in broader digital health solutions such as online scheduling and virtual-first health plan

	Convenience	Experience	Usage	Entry point
Physicians	36	32	10	14

agree that telehealth is more convenient for providers than in-person care	agree telehealth can improve patient experience	expect virtual visits to be 10% of their total visits	have invested in digital front door; only 8% have invested in patient text-messaging platform

Source: McKinsey Physicians Surveys and McKinsey Consumer Surveys, 2020-21   McKinsey & Company

In a recent article from Sanjula Jain, telehealth's Total Addressable Market (TAM) in America is 330M people; from 2019 to 2021, only 84M people used telemedicine. Furthermore, her research showed telemedicine just diversified access to those that already had it. It didn't expand to offer more people access [2].

Recent published results from the American Medical Association based upon the survey of over 2300 doctors, state the vast majority of doctors—85%—are still using telehealth to deliver patient care, and most, 70%, said their organization is motivated to continue using this form of virtual care in their practice [3].

The same example can be made in public health with nutrition. When schools closed down, the food distribution system for kids receiving their meals was completely disrupted. Alternative means to pick up food or have it delivered to homes were created and scaled. Should the new lessons learned and means of distribution be abandoned post pandemic, or is the new way better, more efficient, more effective? I am pleased to share our local food pantry and Meals on Wheels program just received nearly $3.0M to expand the use of the at home delivery platform for clients. This promotes choice as well as home delivery. While some clients still want to come shop at a pantry, the inclusion of multiple distribution channels should be leveraged to reach more people and communities effectively.

Technology provides a viable solution to change the distribution model for healthcare and public health. It does not replace the traditional system, but goals to change at least 50% of the distribution mode of healthcare and public health services, such as education or healthy food, should be set over the next 3 to 5 years. The tools are there. There is

Technology provides a viable solution to change the distribution model for healthcare and public health.

expanding research to prove quality and safety are preserved and even enhanced for many traditional healthcare and public health solutions [4]. There is more data to be reviewed, but the opportunity to validate the clinical efficacy of providing care or social support more effectively with technology as an option, not just face-to-face in a traditional model, and scaling it systemically will most certainly, without question, help address the access issues the traditional systems of both healthcare and public health perpetuate. This, in turn, gives us a viable option and perhaps a more effective remedy on our quest to help solve the equity issues in health and health care.

References:

1) Bestsennyy O, Gilbert G, Harris A, Rost J. Telehealth: a
    quarter-trillion-dollar post-COVID-19 reality? McKinsey.com
    Published July 9, 2021. Accessed March 1, 2022.
    https://www.mckinsey.com/industries/healthcare-
    systems-and-services/our-insights/telehealth-a-quarter-
    trillion-dollar-post-covid-19-reality.

2) Jain S. Telehealth's total addressable market is smaller than
    advertised and continues to decline. Trillianthealth.com.
    Published March 6, 2022. Accessed March 16, 2022.
    https://www.trillianthealth.com/insights/the-
    compass/telehealths-total-addressable-market-smaller-
    than-advertised-and-continues-to-decline.

3) O'Reilly KB. New survey data shows doctors' steadfast
    commitment to Telehealth. AMA-ASSN.org. Published April 1,
    2022. Accessed April 3, 2022. https://www.ama-
    assn.org/practice-management/digital/new-survey-data-
    shows-doctors-steadfast-commitment-telehealth.

4) Telehealth and patient safety during the COVID-19 response.
    Agency for Healthcare Research and Quality.
    PSNET.AHRQ.gov. Published May 14, 2020. Accessed April 2,
    2022. https://psnet.ahrq.gov/perspective/telehealth-and-
    patient-safety-during-covid-19-response.

Opportunity—Framework for Alignment

Together is the Way

THE BARRIER TO date is that we have largely allowed the industry of public health and healthcare to act independently and measure their impact independently. We also do not approach prevention as practice with the same rigor we do medical interventions. We allow for the factors of health to be fragmented to drive subject matter expertise and profit, but we do not require it to be brought back together to be measured and continuously improved. This is the fatal flaw and the fundamental reason why we are not making the progress we need to make. We are allowing ourselves to believe one part is not interconnected to

> **We allow for the factors of health to be fragmented to drive subject matter expertise and profit . . .**

the other. The science and data are diluted in fragments, without bringing back to the whole.

As contemplated earlier in the book, we must figure out how to create a win which allows us to MEET and SURPASS our potential—TOGETHER is the way— and how to stop measuring by just the subcomponents. Unfortunately, our current situation is like proclaiming a football team won the game because the other team forfeited. You can't just ignore the facts that lead up to that moment. The parts have to be summed up or the rules aren't followed and the game isn't complete. How do we create a common scorecard and engage in the same game to help achieve the outcomes together?

The Data Hypothesis

Effectively measuring the SUM of the parts in addition to the parts is the value proposition. Data and analytics are a critical accelerant to bridge the practice of medicine and the practice of public health. The hypothesis: each discipline brings different core competencies to the table therefore utilizing different metrics. Combining the scientific training of a physician and a public health scientist, together overlaid on the same data set, should

> **Effectively measuring the SUM of the parts in addition to the parts is the value proposition.**

yield valid insights on areas of focus to drive not only healthcare but health.

Joining the sciences of public health and medicine around common data sets focused on population health analytics is a critical next step. We have to renew our rigor to hear the story told by the data with a lens of community and individual, together. Instead of taking a tool and finding the problem, let the data illuminate the opportunities, and we apply the appropriate tools to drive an improved outcome. As we validate this in practice, measuring quality, experience, cost and scalability, we can focus on understanding the flow of money and policies which govern the flow of money. Once we have done these things, then we can begin to overlay the science, tools, and outcomes in a way that allows us to effectively question the traditional practice, use data to truly understand the impact, use AI to be more proactive than reactive, and attempt to shift the pot of money where it will drive the most impact. The factors driving health and our definitions of quality provide the roadmap for prioritization and impact, and the funding provides the roadmap for prioritization, implementation, change management, and accelerant/barriers for change. What is measured gets changed, and what is funded gets prioritized and, in turn, drives policy which supports systems. Systems for good. Systems for equity. Systems for positive trending health outcomes for all.

Addressing Equity through Interdependent Systems

While more organizations, including healthcare systems, payers, community organizations, etc., are focused on doing their part to address equity and social determinants of health, if applied in silos we may make assumptions about what individuals need because organizations are applying the tools available. For example, if a system focuses on closing the gap of food insecurity and implements frictionless programs to help access food for its patients, great—for those who have food insecurity as a driving factor. But what if it's housing, violence, or clean air? The expectation is not for organizations to solve this independently; instead, we want to wrap an interdependent system around a person which employs tools to address causal relationships or interdependent variables. And, if there are several, which there more than likely will be, this interdependent system will be able to prioritize.

Healthcare will have a difficult time prioritizing these changes to make it commonplace practice if the financial incentive is still sick care. The momentum has been building since the ACA to incentivize prevention and health. If integrated delivery networks are truly incentivized by outcomes tied to health and prevention, this will be the critical inflection point.

The federal government is pouring money into public health and pandemic preparedness. This is not dissimilar to the money falling from the sky after September 11th, 2001, which was focused on disaster preparedness. If we look back and give ourselves a grade on the measurable impact we made at that moment of crisis, what would we find? Did we buy toys that collected dust and stockpile medications to go unused and expire? Two decades later, is the United States a safer place systemically from disasters and terrorism? Can we prevent these events? Can we react appropriately? How do we measure?

The Bridge

I'll share a story of my involvement in the development of the first of its kind mobile hospital, MED1. Working with Emergency Medicine physicians was one of my greatest fortunes. As I reflect, most of the tangible work I was involved in was spurred by their intelligence and inside view of health and healthcare. Since the Emergency Department is the safety net of the American healthcare system, the team was responsible for saving your life in the most dire of circumstances to serving everything from basic aliments and primary care needs when access and other barriers prevented the full community from reaching primary care providers. One physician in particular had an interest in access to emergency care in the wake of disasters or terrorist events. This was prior to 9/11 so his presentations on attacks fueled by weapons of mass destruction were viewed more as "chicken little" than actual threats. With his innovation and leadership, we received a grant from DHHS to develop the first mobile hospital on wheels—which happened to be rolling out its first training exercise with partnership between the healthcare system, fire, police, and EMS on September 11, 2001.

While field hospitals relying on tent structures had been around for decades, this structure was unique since it was contained in a tractor trailer, with pop out sides to set up ICU beds, treatment bays, and an OR in mere hours. It even had a dental chair! Naively, we thought providing an upgrade to facilities used in times of crisis would be embraced. It was not—and we found ourselves justifying our value compared to the traditional tent structure. Reflecting on the situation at the time, it took leadership from our state and the federal government to pave a path for an asset that could augment and evolve the current solution, not necessarily replace it.

Ironically, while the tractor trailer portion of MED1 provided a significant upgrade and ease of access to clinical tools, it also relied on a tent structure for the less acute to expand the capacity. It was an AND to the current solution, not an OR, and it was very difficult to navigate the common ground. It was difficult because of policy, leadership, and human nature. It took leadership, compromise, and integration to realize the collective full potential. Healthcare and public health. Local, state, and federal government. Individuals and communities—joining forces and finding a better solution together.

Since its inception in 2001, to date MED1 has deployed over twenty times and served hundreds of thousands of people filling the gap of healthcare in dire times. As I reflect on this, the approach to create MED1 was proactive and public health focused—preserving a means to provide healthcare in the wake of disaster. Deployed in a traditional healthcare organization, there were as many who saw its value as those who said it was a waste of funds, time, and energy. It did not fit the mold or align to any of the current regulations at a state or federal level. It provided healthcare services and public health services to people in their most critical time of need. It was the hybrid, a tangible example of the interconnection between healthcare and public health—an asset ready to respond and serve a population, preserving a key factor of health which is healthcare delivery.

MED1 represents the gap—and perhaps the bridge. It's a tool created to respond if a key health factor (hospital/ emergency department) was eliminated from the equation (public health) but only comes to life when the healthcare tool—clinical providers, equipment, medicine, etc.—is added to it, to provide the community in need, and the individuals in the community, with what they needed to maintain or restore health. I can still see the faces of the team—both medical and public health practitioners, the residents, and the other leaders we served with to bring the operation to life. It took us all—federal, state, local, healthcare, public health—to make it happen.

What work needs to be done now to set public health and medicine structure to amplify the funds and the impact? Will we be hard graders or will we not grade at all? Who grades?

There is only ONE word of difference in the definition of public health and medicine and that is populations versus individuals. Both are defined as healing. In medicine, the patient is the individual person. In public health, the patient is the entire community. Let's come together now.

Both/And: Medicine & Public Health Together Conceptual Model

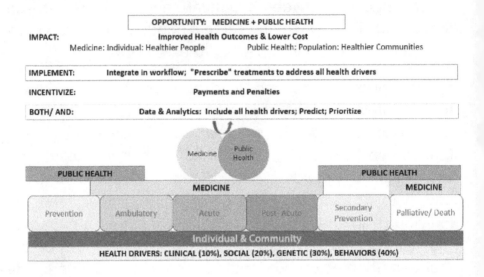

Kaney 2022

THE ASPIRATION:

- The practices of public health and medicine need each other
- Together, we can agree upon a definition for health which is a sum of the disparate parts—including the ultimate goal(s) and metrics of success
- The advancement of tools and tactics to drive health needs to:
    - i. be based upon all health drivers
    - ii. span the full continuum
    - iii. be informed by sciences of both medicine and public health

THE IMPLEMENTATION:

I.   Science has to drive the buy-in for physicians and public health scientists; the buy-in becomes common language speaking to the drivers of health; the drivers of health need to be incentivized by the healthcare and public health system.

II.   This is enabled by medical and public health leadership:

    a. advocating for unification.

    b. utilizing data to understand health across the full continuum, including population and individual insight. The foundation of population health analytics needs to be embraced, embedded in our process of evaluation, and available in widespread accessible education.

III.   The science should inform what is actually driving health and where the priorities are—mutually agreed upon by both professions.

IV.   The business model can be applied at that point to identify resource needs—what is currently spent where, is it adding value (marginal impact) or not, where should it be spent—prevent and eliminate duplication; proactive vs reactive.

V.   The solutions to provide access to the treatment need to be operationalized and scalable in practice. Those accountable for providing the service need to be accountable and held accountable for measuring process for efficiency and outcomes for effectiveness, short and long term.

VI.   Measure, critically think, engage all stakeholders, continuously improve, repeat

Making it a Reality: Medicine and Public Health Together

1) Real-World Population Health Analytics in Community, Public, and Medical Health Systems

Ines M. Vigil, MD, MPH, MBA
Martha L. Sylvia, PhD, MBA, RN

2) Convergence of Diagnostics and Population Health Clinical Lab 2.0

Khosrow R. Shotorbani, MBA, MT
KathleenM. Swanson, MS, RPh
Mark K Fung, MD
PhD, Jill Warrington, MD, PhD
Beth Bailey
Michael J Crossey, MD, PhD

3) It's Not a Flip of The Switch: Piloting Screening for Social Needs in Primary Care

Brisa Urquieta de Hernandez, PhD
Holly Dockery, BS
Iris Cheng MD, FACP
Maria Reese, MPH
Alisahah Jackson, MD

4) Intersection Between Medicine, Physical and Mental Wellbeing, and Public Health

Meghna Patel, MHA

5) Whole Person Index: Now I'm a Believer:

Katie Kaney, DrPH, MBA, FACHE
Carolyn Minnock, MBA

6) Redefining Roles—Payer

Brian Sneve, MPH

Real-World Population Health Analytics in Community, Public, and Medical Health Systems

Ines M. Vigil, MD, MPH, MBA
Martha L. Sylvia, PhD, MBA, RN

Determining What Healthcare Is Needed

WHAT IS THE best and most effective way to identify the health and healthcare needs that exist in a given population? Are these needs different based upon different demographic or medical factors? What are the most important health and social factors to address and in what order or to what degree? How does a health organization know they are successful in reducing health inequity and improving health in a way that impacts the person, the community, the region, and the nation?

Answering the previous questions can be a daunting task and is crucial to ensuring your healthcare organization is well suited and prepared to achieve impact. Population health analytics is a necessary tool in the toolbox to bridge the gap between addressing a population's medical and social needs. The result is a positive impact to the health of individuals, communities, and the healthcare system at large.

Population health analytics, as defined in Drs. Sylvia and Vigil's *Population Health Analytics* textbook, uses a mixture of public health epidemiologic methods and evidence-based practice learnings to identify a population's healthcare needs, uncover the underlying drivers of poor or declining health, and address those drivers of poor health outcomes with a combination of medical and social interventions, while monitoring for impact [1]. It is important for the community, public, and medical health systems to work together to address health and social needs.

Throughout this chapter, we will highlight ways in which population health analytics support the achievement of improved healthcare outcomes. Applying analytics to improve health is best compared to the stages of a relay race that require multiple hand-offs. First, there is a preparation phase that requires an understanding of what data is needed—collecting or aggregating the data in a way that can be used to answer a variety of healthcare questions. Next, there is a starting phase that generates momentum through problem-solving using the data. This is followed by an acceleration phase such that all parts of the healthcare organization can synchronize and have a single source of truth that enables data-driven decision-making and operational efficiency. Finally, there is a results phase that informs any course-correction needed or optimization where appropriate. We will discuss this process, and we will also highlight where barriers exist and ways to avoid or overcome the challenges that lead to failure for many of the healthcare organizations working in this space.

Where is the Data and Who Can Access It?

Gaining access to governed data ready for analytic use is not an easy task to accomplish. It is equally challenging to create and govern data that can be integrated with other relevant data sets to generate population health insights. Gaining access to and creating needed data are perfect examples of why community, public, and medical health systems need to work together to truly address health needs. The following is an example that illustrates a common success and failure of healthcare organizations in accessing and architecting data for use in population health analytics that is neither financially nor operationally feasible for small-to-medium-sized community, public, and medical healthcare organizations.

A small, local, and community-based healthcare system in the mid-Atlantic was interested in understanding the ways in which social factors were preventing individuals from accessing needed care. They chose to focus their resources on a Medicaid benefit-eligible population that accessed care locally, mainly women and children. They were able to collect data on the reasons patients often cancelled scheduled appointments, no-showed to scheduled appointments, or missed needed vaccinations and well-check appointments for their children. They collected the information by surveying their patients, collating the responses into a Word document, and updated the results over time. They analyzed the data with the help of a data analyst who moved the responses to a spreadsheet format. Through this effort they discovered that high temperatures, inclement weather, breakdowns in local transportation routes and vehicles, and the clinic's difficulty with rescheduling appointments in a timely manner, all made it difficult for patients and parents of patients to attend their scheduled appointments and meet their healthcare needs. This resulted in a lack of timely access to needed healthcare. With this finding, the healthcare system was able to partner with local community transportation agencies and allocate resources to create alternative transportation, anticipating the need and ramping up services based upon changes in weather and rerouting of regular local transportation routes.

This scenario is common in healthcare and happens every day across the US. Population health analytics are applied with great success to populations to highlight environmental contributions to health and disease and uncover root causes of healthcare system breakdowns. However, this example is also a healthcare system failure in need of a solution. While the system was able to pull off a one-time root cause analysis across multiple disparate and manually collected and collated data sources, their failure in sustainably accessing and implementing data, developing analytic infrastructure, and using population health models is not thinking ahead to what will be needed in the future. The previous example shows a successful application of population health analytics, but this example also illustrates the failure of the way population health analytics is used in many healthcare organizations because this project is completely unscalable, both operationally and in its impact. In order for this community healthcare system to regularly repeat the analysis for monitoring and communities across the US to benefit from the learnings, the factors preventing individuals from accessing needed care (in this instance, the factors are both environmental and administrative) need to be known and localized by zip code and community, and the data needs to be combined across disparate systems (in this case, weather and scheduling are both important to identifying the cause and enacting the solution). Additionally, public and private partnerships are needed to create effective interventions (in this case, across community health systems and private/public transportation companies).

What organizations have this data available nationally? Does it easily combine together with other supplemental data sets? What is the cost to access and use? Is it affordable for healthcare organizations across the US or are systems destined to create, operate, and maintain data sets and population health data models themselves to identify need and demonstrate impact? Does this render the healthcare industry to only have nominal impact, and does this leave every community, public, and medical healthcare system on their own when it comes to delivering high-value care?

We argue the largest problem to solve in applying population health analytics today is that every health system and community health organization may start from scratch, building their data and analytic infrastructure without the proper expertise or scalability. Most are likely to overspend and over or under architect a solution that ultimately is deemed unusable or ineffective at best. We see this not only across small-to-mid-sized health systems, but also across some regional health systems and health plans. Healthcare is simply spending too much money and setting themselves up for failure trying to accomplish population health analytics on their own. Just think for a moment of the number of resources needed to get from having data to deriving insights to taking action. To have data requires a team of data architects, engineers, scientists, and a technology platform that is unified, governed, transparent in its calculations, inclusions, and exclusions. And that just gets you a dump of data from which to work, a mere starting point. Assuming all goes well and the technical investment bears fruit (which can run as little as a couple of million dollars to tens of millions of dollars over 2 to 5 years' time, depending on the efficiency of healthcare in this space), then you will need more data engineers, scientists, and analysts that deeply understand healthcare operations, workflows, and transaction systems to architect the data into a population health data model to be rendered for analytic use to answer a wide variety of questions across an entire organization's collection of use cases. And if you get this right, then you need a team of clinicians, business leaders, and analysts all trained to work with data to ask the right questions, apply the most appropriate analytic model or calculation, and map it to the most effective and impactful intervention. Assuming this goes well and you have a plethora of insights and proposed interventions, you will then need a highly skilled operations team to apply the intervention to the population identified to receive the most benefit, monitor for impact, remove barriers, and track results.

This does not seem possible or reasonable. Yet we have seen firsthand the tragedy of many healthcare organizations attempting to master the feat above. We have been brought into organizations to fix the data, people, and process chaos made, and, on multiple occasions, we have relayed the bad news to C-suite leaders of the sunk cost that neither delivered value nor can be recovered without massive new investment.

As an alternative to this fruitless investment, we propose that most healthcare organizations NOT become their very own analytics and technology platform company, further distracting it from accomplishing their healthcare delivery mission, but instead begin to treat the collection, availability, aggregation, governance, transparency, and analytic use of data as a commodity, accessible by all and a universal source of truth within and across organizations.

One solution to the overwhelming endeavor and possible failure of building it yourself is to look to the handful of data analytics and technology companies that exist today that are already working to bring these disparate datasets together, providing healthcare organizations with an existing, robust, governed data set that is ready for analytic use and large enough data assets to reach statistical significance, enabling healthcare organizations to instead focus resources and efforts on solving for the healthcare needs identified through the use of these solutions. If you are a healthcare CEO, CFO, or CMO, ask yourself this question, 'Should I really be dedicating my organization's time and resources to building something that may work but not meet the need at best and at worst not work at all?' If you are a healthcare data engineer, scientist, analyst working in a care delivery or local/regional health plan organization, ask yourself this question, 'Am I making a positive contribution to healthcare by building a solution that may never meet the standards for accuracy, transparency, governance, or statistical significance warranted to enable clinicians and administrators to take action with confidence of doing no harm?'.

We are not advocating every healthcare organization eliminate its technical and analytic workforce. We do, however, advocate for organizations to buy what can be built better by others whose expertise and focus is on this task day-in and day-out, and to repurpose your existing staff on developing new data sources and data sets that can be incorporated into existing purchased data and infrastructure and translating the data into insights and action to be more easily adopted by care delivery teams and administrative leaders. We also advocate for reallocating funding to add resources to develop an organization of people, processes, and culture that know what to do with the insights derived from data and how to apply it, to whom, and to a defined intended end result, absent of harm.

Creating the Data Healthcare Needs

Are you a healthcare organization that wants to innovate, make a positive health contribution to your community and that of others, or have demonstrable impact on health nationally? If you answered yes to these questions, consider making a contribution that can be aggregated across all other like organizations' contributions by scanning your organization's initiatives to gather what has truly worked to improve health in your local, regional, and national populations and start to develop a data set, identification algorithms, and intervention leading and lagging monitoring measures that truly enable a scalable solution to be developed. This is a truly worthy use and application of your teams of data-oriented technology and analytic resources and advances healthcare into the 21st century, with the potential to make a more demonstrable impact on improving health outcomes across the US.

It is important for the stakeholders in healthcare to capitalize on one another's strengths and strengthen one another's weaknesses in the process. If our recommendation becomes reality, where the aggregation, governance, operation, and maintenance of data assets and population health data models are owned by nationally-based analytics and technology companies and delivered to healthcare organizations across the US, could the following also be fulfilled:

- Payers or the government can subsidize or cover the cost of healthcare organizations accessing a universal source of truth for healthcare data.
- A set of financially and scientifically vetted code standards can be adopted and applied to healthcare organizations wishing to innovate with existing data or contribute new data.
- Healthcare organizations can refocus their existing resources on creating new and innovative solutions, interventions, and inventions from the insights gleaned from this universal data asset.
- Payers and providers can truly partner to solve the crisis of poor healthcare outcomes and unsustainable healthcare finances.

It is an equally challenging task to create a data asset, identification criteria, leading and lagging monitoring measures that identify an opportunity mapped to an evidence-based intervention aimed at improving health outcomes. Nevertheless, community, public, and medical healthcare organizations are perfectly suited to succeed in this work. You hold within your organizations the ability, willingness, and nimbleness to enact and track progress quickly, fail fast, realize impact firsthand, and iterate to identify what set of interventions, processes, and programs work best, tailored to the unique characteristics of the people and communities you serve. By creating impactful protocols, interventions, inventions that can be shared with health systems across the US, you position yourself to create your largest possible contribution to the improvement of health for all. You would also have access to the contributions of others, thereby propagating mutual success.

There is some work to do to create a data asset, identification criteria, leading and lagging monitoring measures, and this all assumes you come to the table with a sizeable, robust, complete, governed, and transparent data set. It also assumes that you have access to a set of analytic software tools to analyze the data, and a team of clinicians, business leaders, and analysts trained to ask questions of data, develop or match to evidence-based interventions, or design benefits and programs with impact.

See where we are going with this? There is so much work to do after having the data that is perfectly suited to advancing your care delivery mission, your teams' skill sets, and your resource prioritization process that will bring forward pockets of scalable innovation with the potential to leapfrog healthcare into this century and beyond. The image that follows captures the complexity of the individual, behavioral, infrastructure, administrative, and systematic factors at play when developing scalable healthcare solutions. We propose that healthcare organizations focus their time and resources on designing and applying evidence-based interventions and programs tailored to the unique needs of your populations, and we offer a little guidance and a framework to follow [2].

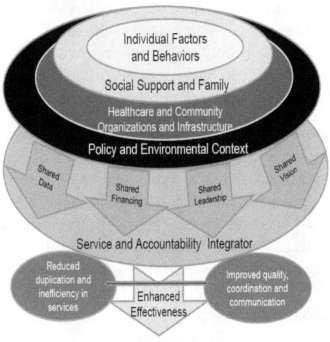

Sherry, MK; Wolff, JL; Ballreich, J; DuGoff, E; Davis, K;Anderson, G. Bridging the Silos of Service Delivery for High-Need, High-Cost Patients. Journal of Population Health Management. Online before print: March 23, 2016

A Little Guidance and a Framework to Follow

Every organization embarking on the journey to delivering value-based care needs a population health framework to guide the thought process, define value, and ensure the complexities highlighted in the previous conceptual model are addressed. Finding and addressing root causes of worsening health outcomes requires scientific know-how and an understanding of how people's behaviors influence how they care for themselves and others. We developed the population health analytics framework below out of a need for a step-wise approach to applying population health and data-driven decision-making. We identified this need after working across several payers and providers of varying size across the US who were entering into value-based care arrangements without a clear understanding of their populations' needs, root causes of health and disease, and the opportunities to improve care delivery, quality, and affordability. This framework also supports a stronger partnership between communities, the public, and medicine. Figure 1 depicts for each phase the process, the purpose, and the analytics needed. Ideally the phases are undertaken in successive order for each question asked of your data. Four components are critical when engaging in analytics as part of a medicine and public health partnership including describing populations, developing and implementing targeting algorithms, developing and measuring process and outcome metrics, and monitoring and optimizing interventions.

Defining a population tailored to the problem being addressed is the first step to improving outcomes and is the product of the assess phase. For instance, when the problem to address is improving glucose control in people with diabetes served by a rural community center, the population may be defined in data terms as all people with the health condition diabetes, living within a certain distance from the community center, and perhaps with a history of poor glucose control. It's also important to understand the population's needs and determine root causes for poor glycemic control, including demographics such as age, gender, and race/ethnicity; access to healthcare and community services such as identification of the primary care provider, health insurance status, community services participation; socioeconomic factors such as income source and level, living situation, family support for chronic conditions; and more. The need for integrated social and medical data from the community center, the medical system, and other sources becomes readily apparent when looking to uncover root causes of disease, disability, and health.

Figure 1: The Population Health Process and Associated Analytics

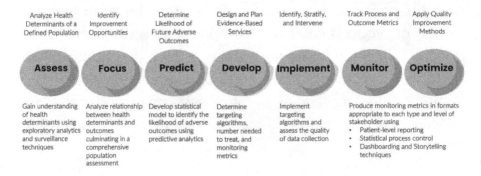

Reproduced from Sylvia M. Introduction to population health analytics. In: *Population Health Management Learning Series.* Forestvue Healthcare Solutions;2020 [3].

Once populations are defined, described, and root causes of problems identified, interventions can be designed or applied to address root causes and mitigate poor health outcomes. In order to intervene, a list of people with the associated risk factors identified as root causes is needed. This is where targeting algorithms come in. A targeting algorithm lays out the criteria by which a person is identified as having one or more risks that would qualify them for an intervention, stratified to match them to the intervention from which they will receive the most benefit, and segmented or tailored to ensure the intervention will meet individual needs. Using the findings from the population description, a list of people with identified needs is produced, mapped to an intervention from which they are likely to receive and provide benefit [1]. Figure 2 shows an example of a simplified targeting algorithm, directing people to appropriate interventions, based on their unique characteristics and needs.

Figure 2: Targeting Algorithm Example

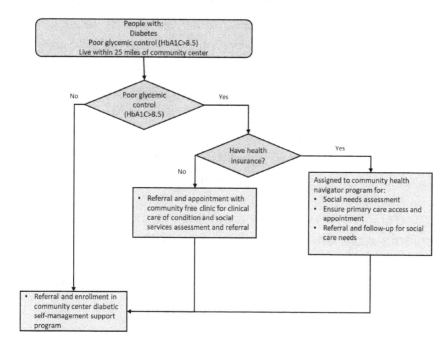

Reproduced from Sylvia M. Stratifying and segmenting populations. In: *Population Health Management Learning Series.* Forestvue Healthcare Solutions; 2020 [4].

Once interventions are designed and appropriately targeted to the people who need them, the next step is to determine the degree to which the interventions are working. *Are people receiving all program components and when they do, are the intended outcomes achieved?* This is where metrics, monitoring, and optimization become critical to the success of population health strategies. Our guidance is to measure both process and outcomes simultaneously to ensure the specific details of the intervention are being implemented as designed, and to what degree the intervention results in the intended outcome. In the example in Figure 2, process measures might include the percentage of people who were without health insurance who were seen for diabetes at the community clinic or the percentage of people with good glucose control who enrolled in a self-management support program. Outcomes measure whether the ultimate result, usually in the category of health outcomes, experience of care, or cost/utilization of care, also known as The Triple Aim objectives, is achieved. The outcome measure of interest in the example in Figure 2 is the percentage of people with diabetes living within 25 miles of the community center who achieve improved glucose control (HbA1C<8.5).

Once measures are determined, monitoring and optimization techniques are employed. Monitoring is the activity of putting the measure results into a format that can be visualized over time. We recommend using a run chart which contains the results of the measure (usually monthly) and a median line across all time intervals as a reference point or a more sophisticated statistical process control chart (SPC) which also displays the results of the measure with the mean value and control limits. Run and SPC charts can be established to determine the degree to which intervention processes are running as they should and if the intervention is impacting outcomes [5]. Figure 3 is an example of an SPC chart.

Optimization is an opportunity to course correct for any challenges, barriers, or behaviors not originally anticipated that may be negatively effecting your process and outcomes performance. We recommend using a quality improvement process such as Plan, Do, Study, Act. Stakeholders are identified at the initiation of the intervention and include clinical, administrative, analytic, and operations leaders. The group meets daily, weekly, or monthly depending on the intervention to review results, identify areas for improvement, strategize action steps, execute tactics, and monitor process and outcomes measures [1].

Figure 3: Statistical Process Control Chart Example

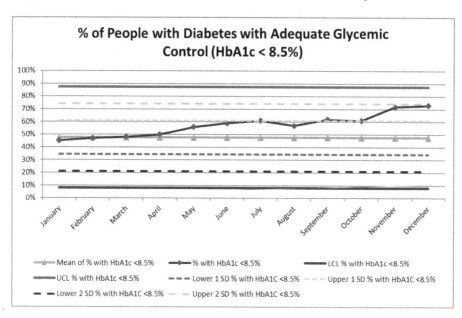

Reproduced from Sylvia M. Statistical process control for monitoring population health interventions. In: *Population Health Management Learning Series.* Forestvue Healthcare Solutions; 2020 [6].

Stacking Hands across Community, Public, and Medical Health Systems

The systems needed to transact, compile, normalize, govern, and surface data to support population health analytics and address root causes of health, disease, and disability is multifactorial and complex. This is all the more reason for community, public, and medical health systems to partner together to secure access to readied data and robust analytic solutions so you can leapfrog into figuring out what your populations need, what barriers exist to accessing needed care, and what interventions have the most potential impact to improving health outcomes. Figure 4 depicts the intricacies of the complex and multifactorial data and analytics system.

Figure 4: Structures and Processes of a System Supporting Integrated Analytics

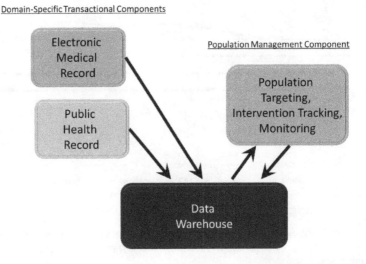

Adapted from Cuddeback JK, Fisher DW. Information technology. In: Nash et al. *Population Health Management*, 2nd Edition. Jones and Bartlett Learning; 2016 [7].

To illustrate the complexity, on the left of the diagram in Figure 4, transaction systems are shown. These are the systems that clinicians and public health practitioners use in their interactions or encounters with individual patients. This is where individual data points, collected at the point of care are entered, decision support is used to guide clinical care, and patient portals are used to exchange information with patients and caregivers. Integrated medicine and public health transactional systems are usually unique to each entity. Providers across multiple health systems will each have their own electronic medical record, and public health providers will also have their own unique transactional systems.

To the right of Figure 4, the population management component is relatively new and important for integrated medical and public health systems, and this component works best when shared between public health and medical entities. The Parkland Center for Clinical Innovation (PCCI) describes a model population health management component

> ... **the population management component is relatively new and important for integrated medical and public health systems, and this component works best when shared between**

where a transactional system is unified across community organizations and medical care. In this model, the shared transactional system includes notifications, secured messaging, referral management, scheduling, document management, decision support, eligibility management, and reporting. The systems are designed under the direction of a multi-disciplinary stakeholder oversight group [8].

At the bottom of the diagram, data collected in the transactional systems are organized in a data warehouse which is an environment that relates data in a logical way in support of the ability to store this data over time and query this data for analytic purposes. A data warehouse can organize and store data from multiple source systems, group and contextualize data for analytic purposes, and send processed data back to transactional systems for decision support purposes [1]. Individual providers and public health entities usually have some type of data warehouse functionality, but that is not always the case. Smaller healthcare organizations with few resources may not have a data warehouse. In these cases, reporting and analysis of data is done directly out of the transactional system. Population health and value-based care best practice, however, recommends a data warehouse for these functions so that transactional systems are not compromised by querying and analytic processes.

What are community, public, and medical systems to do who can neither build nor individually afford the data needed? We propose what is needed is twofold. First is the partnering of community, public, and medical systems across a defined geographic region to bring forward a unified interest and ability to leverage data for the good of the community, each contributing what they can to a budget and accessing much more than they would be able to individually. Second is for private and government payers to subsidize the medical and care delivery community to share in the cost burden of data and analytic solutions, ensuring a unified source of truth across a region and a partnership of efforts across communities all served by those operating in the defined region. An integrated medicine and public health system, a shared defined data set, a unified data warehouse, and a single source of truth are ideal for supporting key competencies in population health and value-based care. Success in an integrated community/ public/medicine health system analytics program requires transactional and population health to be integrated into a universal and robust data warehouse. When seeking the ideal shared data set and analytic solutions, it is important to ensure that the following core competencies exist:

> **An integrated medicine and public health system, a shared defined data set, a unified data warehouse, and a single source of truth are ideal for supporting key competencies in population health and value-based care.**

- Existing data assets that represent claims, SDoH, medical, and supplemental data.
- Breadth and depth of data coverage across existing data assets nationally.
- Mechanisms for querying the data to identify persons eligible for intervention and ability to create targeted lists for intervention teams.
- Mechanisms for sharing data including the secure transfer of data and shared data storage space.
- Person-level detail and management of individual people must be matched across data sets with the ability to eliminate duplication of the same person and ensure that all qualified people are captured in merged data sets [1].
- Universal and appropriate use of definitions of key concepts in data terms, methods for grouping data, definitions of

process and outcome metrics including denominators and numerators in data terms, methods for determining successful outcomes (benchmarking, targets, using comparison groups), and, above all, transparency in all data calculations and applied methods.

Meeting this basic set of competencies ensures that data is sufficient to be accurate and relevant, data can be shared across entities, individuals can be identified across data sets, and that entities share a common set of data, grouping, and metric definitions.

How to Contribute Value by Collecting and Structuring Data for Analytics

The greatest advantage that community, public, and medical health systems possess is the ability to interact with people and identify information impactful to their health that would otherwise go unrecognized. As healthcare evolves and population health initiatives grow to support value-based care delivery, so does the need for relevant information that traditional healthcare transaction systems do not collect. Important considerations for data collection in community, public, and medical health systems partnerships include the decision to collect data automatically as part of existing electronic data collection systems, to devise new data collection systems that collect data electronically, or to devise new data systems that collect data manually. If at all possible,

> **The greatest advantage that community, public, and medical health systems possess is the ability to interact with people and identify information impactful to their health that would otherwise go unrecognized.**

needed data should be extracted from existing electronic data collection systems. This is the most feasible, economical, and timely manner of data collection because it is a repurposing of data that is already being collected. If data does not already exist for the use-case at hand, a new data collection system must be designed. Electronic data collection is the most feasible because of scalability, ease of administration, timeliness, and the ability to easily track responses. The least desirable method of collecting needed data is manually because it is labor intensive, difficult to administer and track, and is most likely to result in data quality errors [5].

It is also important to understand the value of data standardization for interoperability or the ability to exchange and use data across computer systems. Generally, the higher the level of interoperability, the higher the value, scalability, and functionality of the data. Additionally, the more interoperable a data set is, the less likely it will disappear from existence due to its owner transitioning out of the organization or getting lost in a sea of corporate documents saved on a work drive. At the foundational level of interoperability, interconnectivity requirements are met for systems to securely give and receive data. The movement of a patient record in PDF format between two electronic medical records is at this basic level of interoperability. At the next level, the exchange of data uses the same format, syntax, and organization. An example would be the exchange of a data set with rows and columns where the columns are in the same order with each exchange, each column of data has a set format, and each column represents a discrete concept. Exchange of data files from organizations like CMS to health plans use this level of interoperability. At the next level, data elements have standardized definitions, value sets, and coding vocabularies resulting in shared meaning of data between systems. At the final level of interoperability data governance and policies as well as social, legal, and organizational considerations facilitate the secure, seamless, and timely communication and use of data between organizations [9]. Table 1 shows an example of data exchange at each level of interoperability using allergies as an example.

Table 1: Exchange of Allergy Information at Incremental Levels of Interoperability

Level	Example of Data Exchange
Foundational	A patient note in the form of a PDF includes the sentence, "patient is allergic to mushrooms."
Level 2	A data set with a row for each patient and a column titled "allergies" is exchanged. For the same patient as in the foundational level, the term "mushrooms" is entered in the allergy field.
Level 3	The data exchange in Level 2 includes a coding system used by both entities in the exchange that numbers "mushrooms" as a "3." For the same patient in Level 2 using the same data set structure, the code "3" is entered in the field "allergies."
Level 4	There exists one data governance committee across both entities that assigns stewardship over data and oversees standardized definitions, models, and coding vocabularies.

Demonstrate Your Value and Make the Most Impactful Contribution Simultaneously

Your unique ability to partner with other like healthcare organizations with similar goals, the nimbleness of your operations to pivot resources and content to deliver meaningful care, and your ability to collect information needed to tailor care to the unique characteristics to address care gaps to improve health outcomes are all needed to succeed in population health analytics, population and public health interventions, and value-based care arrangements. When focused on identifying what works to improve health outcomes, creating new and novel data assets, identification algorithms mapped to evidence-based interventions, and process and outcome measures with defined populations, thresholds, and expected results are all valuable contributions to advancing healthcare in the US community, public health, and medical health systems are uniquely positioned and organized to deliver. This requires partnership, already existing data and analytics tools, and a penchant for innovation.

In exchange for the valuable data collection, novel data assets, and interoperability, you can ask your private and government payers to subsidize the cost of already existing claims and medical and supplemental data provided to you by several existing data and analytics technology companies, creating a mutual WIN and springboarding your organization's ability to create even more value now and into the future.

This chapter highlights what it takes for the industry as a whole to recognize what they can and should build, what they should buy, and where they should partner to synergize efforts and impact. We emphasize the need for healthcare organizations to partner to capitalize on one another's strengths, using the most efficient analytic tools and strategies to address the needs across shared communities. We believe community, public, and medical health systems are uniquely qualified to create novel data assets tied to action and further drive results in a way that addresses the unique needs and acknowledges their unique characteristics. By understanding how data sources are architected, can be made to be interoperable, are unique and tied to value, your organization can make a significant impact to improved health outcomes for not only your population but also for others across the US. So please skip the hard and laborious work of collating, aggregating, and governing data sets that have little relevance or accuracy, skip combining it with transactional data and building a questionable data warehouse. You have the ability to reallocate your existing right set of people, skills, processes, and resources to create, maintain, and transfer novel data and with it you can build a future of action and impact that propels us all into a healthier future. To what degree are you willing to do it?

References:

1) Sylvia M, Vigil I. *Population Health Analytics*. Jones and Bartlett Learning;2022.

2) Sherry MK, Wolff JL, Ballreich J, DuGoff E, Davis K, Anderson G. Bridging the silos of service delivery for high-need, high-cost patients. *Journal of Population Health Management*. 2016;19(6):421-428.

3) Sylvia M. Introduction to population health analytics. In: *Population Health Management Learning Series*. Forestvue Healthcare Solutions;2020.

4) Sylvia M. Stratifying and segmenting populations. In: *Population Health Management Learning Series*. Forestvue Healthcare Solutions; 2020.

5) Sherry M, Sylvia M. Ongoing monitoring. In: Sylvia M & Terhaar M, eds. *Clinical Analytics and Data Management for the DNP*. Springer Publishing;2023.

6) Sylvia M. Statistical process control for monitoring population health interventions. In: *Population Health Management Learning Series*. Forestvue Healthcare Solutions; 2020.

7) Cuddeback JK, Fisher DW. Information technology. In: Nash et al. *Population Health Management*, 2nd Edition. Jones and Bartlett Learning; 2016.

8)   Kosel K, Miff S. *Building Connected Communities of Care.*
CRC Press;2020. Healthcare Information and Management
Society (HIMSS). Interoperability in Healthcare.
https://www.himss.org/resources/interoperability-
healthcare. Published 2022. Accessed August 11, 2022.

9)   Healthcare Information and Management Society (HIMSS).
Interoperability in Healthcare.
https://www.himss.org/resources/interoperability-
healthcare. Published 2022. Accessed August 11, 2022.

Convergence of Diagnostics and Population Health: Clinical Lab 2.0

Khosrow R. Shotorbani, MBA, MT
KathleenM. Swanson, MS, RPh
Mark K Fung, MD
PhD, Jill Warrington, MD, PhD
Beth Bailey
Michael J Crossey, MD, PhD

Background

THE COVID-19 PANDEMIC has illustrated how today's healthcare environment and current delivery models are ill-equipped to adequately address community health and public safety. Through the process of "test, trace, treat," the pandemic has moved public health and clinical diagnostics to the center of attention; the partnership between these two healthcare verticals has collectively informed healthcare policy, care delivery, and community actions. Still, a multitude of new opportunities exist, emphasizing the necessity for clinical laboratories of the future to step out of their traditional healthcare vertical and develop new active partnerships to support community health and establish a common mission of embracing epidemiologic and population health principles [1].

Similar to the objectives of clinical laboratories, population health, defined as "the health outcomes of a group of individuals, including the distribution of such outcomes within the group" [2], aims to serve both individuals and populations. Population health considers the social, economic, biologic, and environmental determinants to shape the health of an entire population and to promote measurable improvement in the health of a defined population [2, 3] by incorporating four interacting concepts or pillars: chronic care management, quality and safety, public health, and health policy [3]. Embracing population health principles will require laboratories to collaborate with health systems, state and local health departments, primary care providers, information technology, and policy makers.

This chapter, which is based on an article previously published in *Population Health Management* [4], proposes an advanced role for the clinical laboratory as a key partner for health outcomes and public safety. The model, described as the *Future Role of Clinical Lab in Population Health*, promotes the clinical laboratory as pivotal in the formation of a *comprehensive data* and *clinical action platform* to facilitate improved community health. The four dimensions of the Quadruple Aim—better outcomes, lower total cost of care,

> **This chapter . . . proposes an advanced role for the clinical laboratory as a key partner for health outcomes and public safety.**

improved patient experience, and provider experience that optimizes health system performance—serve as the core of this model. Its components work synergistically to create an ecosystem that can be applied in any community or country to promote population health management [5, 6].

As evidenced by previous work, the Clinical Lab 2.0 movement serves as an ideal conduit for delivery on the principles of this model. As first published in 2017 in *Academic Pathology* with an article entitled *Improving American Healthcare through "Clinical Lab 2.0." A Project Santa Fe Report* [7], the role of the Project Santa Fe Foundation (PSFF) and the Clinical Lab 2.0 movement has been to provide thought leadership and assistance to develop the evidence base for the future valuation of clinical laboratory services. Through evolution of the clinical laboratory business model, laboratories can move from a commodity with transactional delivery of test results for sick care defined as "Clinical Lab 1.0" to an integrative component of value-based care providing clinical insights defined as "Clinical Lab 2.0" [7]. PSFF today actively supports organizations globally to demonstrate these principles. Publications describing Clinical Lab 2.0 concepts have highlighted the laboratory's role in population health and chronic disease management in support of value-based healthcare. Authors have demonstrated how laboratory data can contribute to clinical decision support and actionable patient data [8,9], provide value for health plans monitoring chronic conditions such as diabetes [10], and apply real-time laboratory analytics to support disease surveillance [11]. These examples describe how the laboratory can create clinical strategies for early identification of disease, monitor chronic conditions, and support new methods of providing disease management with clinical interventions that can mitigate clinical and financial risk.

Clinical Lab 2.0 can augment the reactionary "test, trace, treat" process by promoting early risk identification in chronic diseases and identify opportunities for active intervention prior to hospitalization, leading to downstream cost avoidance for most chronic and costly conditions. This hidden but measurable value from proactive laboratory insights allows for the recognition of illness before it has advanced and monitoring of diseases at the earlier stages of progression. For example, laboratory information can be used to identify acute kidney injury even when the patient is within a normal creatinine clearance range.

The application of Clinical Lab 2.0 concepts described for chronic diseases can be adapted for high prevalence infectious diseases, including COVID-19. Application of the Clinical Lab 2.0 concepts to support the COVID-19 pandemic has the potential to extend collaboration with public health outside of the traditional reporting of infectious disease case counts. In this new, advanced role, the laboratory could serve as an essential resource for population health and public safety. If engaged, laboratories can find themselves as health professionals who are first to know and first to respond. Laboratories could provide predictive data analytics and facilitate clinical services to limit the spread of disease, re-engage those needing healthcare after the pandemic, and avoid unnecessary expenses to the healthcare system both now and after the pandemic.

Future Role of Clinical Lab 2.0 in Population Health

Using the Clinical Lab 2.0 concepts previously mentioned, the Future Role of Clinical Lab 2.0 in Population Health (Figure 1) was created. Key features of the model include consumer activation through shared decision making and use of social determinants, a data lens for both the individual consumer and the larger population, and development of new health-care delivery models that include primary care and chronic disease management.

> ... the potential value of the clinical laboratory doesn't end at the time of the test result, rather this is where the laboratory value begins to be realized.

While the model is technology agnostic, it recognizes the importance of data analytics, and even artificial intelligence (AI), for success and scalability. This position paper starts with the following premise: 1) the potential value of the clinical laboratory doesn't end at the time of the test result, rather this is where the laboratory value begins to be realized; and 2) the clinical laboratory can support community health by providing risk stratification, closing gaps in care, and facilitating clinical interventions, thus leading to improved outcomes and cost avoidance.

With the Quadruple Aim at the core, the ecosystem illustrated in this model includes four interlocking components working together to leverage the role of the clinical laboratory to support population health: Engage, Test, Analyze, and Partner.

These four elements provide a roadmap on how to fully leverage the clinical laboratory and optimize the health of our patients, families, and communities. Figure 1 illustrates the synergistic interplay of these components:

1) **Engage**: Consumer Activation
2) **Test**: Clinical Lab 1.0
3) **Analyze**: Clinical Lab 2.0
4) **Partner**: Community Health

Figure 1: Future Role of Clinical Lab 2.0 in Population Health

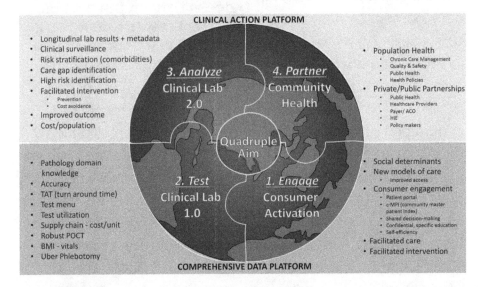

Component 1: Engage—Consumer Activation Utilizing Determinants of Health

The foundation of the model begins with the engaged health consumer. Consumer activation identifies the importance of recognizing and leveraging determinants of health to design care models of the future and promote improved access to care during the early stages of illness [12]. Information and tools available to consumers include the individual's personal data transformed into actionable insights, tools to address their determinants of health, and population health insights such as gaps in care and comorbidities. Increasingly, patients will have an opportunity to directly access their own laboratory test results in real-time, allowing for self-care and wellness decisions. Patients should ultimately be connected to a community master patient index (c-MPI) to promote an integrated consumer driven healthcare experience and inform their healthcare decision making. Mechanisms to engage consumers may include comprehensive care patient portals and laboratory result interpretation.

Consumer activation can also create opportunities to improve a patient's access to care and foster collaborations to facilitate care using insights created with laboratory data. Laboratorians support consumer activation by directly interacting with patients and providers. Providers benefit from the lab's role in consumer activation when they have real time access to patient results presented in a meaningful and historical fashion. Examples of this in the COVID-19 environment include engaging patients to quarantine when needed or to continue routine healthcare with confidence during the pandemic for preexisting conditions.

*Actions laboratories can implement to support Component 1,
Consumer Activation:*

- *Identify data sources for core determinants of health available internally and externally such as comorbid health conditions, gaps in care, and social determinants of health.*
- *Identify mechanisms to support consumer interactions with the healthcare ecosystem and enhance care delivery.*
- *Identify and implement mechanisms such as patient portals or state wide health information exchanges (HIE) to promote shared data and consumer decision making.*
- *Establish the laboratory as a resource in Community Health Needs Assessments (CHNA) as outlined by Affordable Care Act*
- *Create mechanisms with members of the healthcare community to improve patient's access to care using laboratory data.*

Component 2: Test—Clinical Lab 1.0

The second component of the model's foundation includes the laboratory's backbone of essential healthcare services: the timely delivery of accurate test results with high sensitivity and specificity, or Clinical Lab 1.0. Fundamental attributes of Clinical Lab 1.0 are based in pathology and clinical laboratory science domain knowledge and represent the current focus of clinical laboratories to produce six sigma high quality results for clinical treatment decisions. Other attributes of Clinical Lab 1.0 include appropriate test utilization to ensure the right test, at the right time, for the right patient and supply chain management to reduce cost per test. Finally, Clinical Lab 1.0 recognizes the laboratory's many and diverse patient touchpoints, providing abundant patient and data access opportunities. Additional services in the Clinical Lab 1.0 component include point of care testing (POCT), the collection of biometrics and other clinical data, and delivery of phlebotomy services in the clinic or the patient's home. An example of this with COVID-19 includes the provision of POCT in congregate care living facilities to protect high risk individuals. Importantly, all Clinical 1.0 activities build a longitudinal record of measurable and actionable laboratory data.

Actions laboratories can implement to support Component 2, Clinical Lab 1.0:

- *Implement a robust POCT process to support clinical decisions at the point of care and assure POCT results are captured as part of the electronic data or master patient index (eEMPI).*
- *Measure and report changes in measured deltas or changes in key clinical assays indicative of biological change or worsening or improvement of a clinical condition.*
- *Capture additional information such as biometrics to augment data mining for risk stratification when providing outpatient phlebotomy services.*
- *Implement phlebotomy services that come to the patient's geographic location (Uber phlebotomy) to promote proactive care and patient convenience in order to close gaps in care and support ongoing chronic disease management.*
- *Identify opportunities for telehealth-based care delivery specimen collection through shipping services.*

Foundation: Comprehensive Data Platform

The activities within the first two components of the model, Consumer Activation and Clinical Lab 1.0, create a foundational *comprehensive diagnostic data platform* that provides rich predictive and prescriptive data for the lab's pivotal role in optimizing population health management.

Component 3: Analyze - Clinical Lab 2.0

Atop the foundation of consumer engagement and laboratory testing, the third component of the model is Clinical Lab 2.0 insights. Clinical Lab 2.0 insights allow laboratories to harness aggregate longitudinal lab data with a patient-centric view to identify, stratify, track, and monitor patients. Uses of longitudinal data to develop actionable insights for members of the healthcare

> **Clinical Lab 2.0 insights allow laboratories to harness aggregate longitudinal lab data with a patient-centric view to identify, stratify, track, and monitor patients.**

ecosystem (provider, patient, payer, health system, public health) include identification of clinical risk from comorbidities, gaps in care, and facilitation of healthcare interventions using the laboratory's infrastructure.

These actionable insights require several fundamental ingredients: understanding of disease prevalence and the associated clinical and financial burden, active laboratory leadership and lab medicine's domain knowledge, and longitudinal laboratory data (Figure 2). Laboratorians possess significant domain knowledge linking laboratory data to disease diagnostics and progression. Longitudinal laboratory data includes not just laboratory results for individualized patients but also metadata gathered from laboratory orders. Examples of metadata include geographic data such as county or zip code, gender, age, location of healthcare services (ie., emergency room, urgent care, outpatient provider, hospital), concomitant health conditions both chronic and acute, and social determinants of health. This untapped information offers the advantage of having near zero latency and being regularly updated as a result of frequent patient touchpoints with the laboratory. This combination of longitudinal laboratory data and geographic and demographic metadata is of particular value when shared in partnership with community health and public health partners.

Clinical Lab 2.0 insights may also include the provision of more actionable and understandable laboratory results for the provider, patient, and caregivers. This supports consumer activation by empowering patients in their own chronic disease management. Clinical Lab 2.0 insights, especially coupled with patient activation, have the potential to improve clinical and financial outcomes and decrease disease burden. The value proposition of Clinical Lab 2.0 insights is most notable when used to support early identification of a condition prior to disease progression.

When applied to COVID-19, these components can be used to proactively stratify patients at risk after testing positive, identify patients needing isolation and quarantine, provide follow up for post-COVID care, and support healthcare systems to deliver care to non-COVID patients thereby supporting revenue generation.

Figure 2: Clinical Lab 2.0 Model

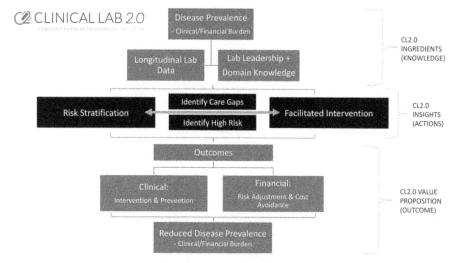

Actions laboratories can implement to support Component 3, Clinical Lab 2.0:

- *Capture longitudinal lab data in a patient centric enterprise Master Patient Index (e-MPI) to support data sharing and interoperability of patient results and provide insights through longitudinal data*
- *Implement processes or technologies that assure timely data acquisition to provide near real-time actionable information at the time of care*
- *Implement operating strategies to build data analytics for identification of gaps in care and risk stratification of high-prevalence and high-cost diseases using internal or external technology to create dashboards, interpretative results, and trend analysis (as used for quality improvement)*

- *Work with other health professionals and administrators to develop and facilitate clinical interventions focused on early care management to slow disease progression (such as acute kidney injury) using laboratory insights*
- *Align laboratory efforts with organizational priorities to improve patient outcomes and reduce financial risk*
- *Engage organizational leadership outside the laboratory to identify opportunities where the laboratory can impact financial and clinical risk*
- *Measure how laboratory insights have changed the total cost of care*

Component 4: Partner - Community Health

The last component of the model recognizes the importance of partnerships with the key stakeholders of population health to create the strategies and policies needed in this new era of healthcare. Alignment with these stakeholders is essential to establish the environment to make the model effective. To support community health, the laboratory must align with the four pillars of population health: chronic care management, quality and safety, public health, and health policy [3]. Additionally, harmonizing with the recently updated ten essential public health services [13] including those focused on assessment and policy development could support implementation. Partnerships with community health leverage the lab's existing relationships, Clinical Lab 1.0 testing results, and Clinical Lab 2.0 insights from data analytics and data platforms. Additional public and private collaborations can also be an important part of this component with providers, payers, and health information exchanges (HIEs).

Actions laboratories can implement to support Component 4, Community Health:

- *Establish an ongoing dialogue with local public health professionals to develop a clinical collaboration supporting a common vision*
- *Establish clinical surveillance of high-prevalence diseases using available geographic location data and other metadata*
- *Identify potential policies addressing early detection and intervention of chronic conditions such as diabetes*

Clinical Action Platform

By connecting components three and four, Clinical Lab 2.0, and community health, a *clinical action platform* can be created for new proactive initiatives and care algorithms by the healthcare ecosystem. The clinical action platform can impact both the larger population and subgroups of patients including those with high-risk medical diagnosis and living conditions. The domain knowledge of laboratory medicine, its vast patient touchpoints, physical proximity to patients, and real-time insights all support the *clinical action platform* and allow the laboratory to be a catalyst for population health leading to positive clinical and financial outcomes. The *clinical action platform* completes the circle, leading back to the consumer, and the need for consumer engagement in order to develop and deliver coordinated interdisciplinary interventions. When applied to COVID-19, for example, the laboratory can assist in the appropriate and efficient identification, risk-stratification, isolation, and quarantine of patients.

Call to Action

Laboratories and community health groups can become active participants in the design and implementation of future delivery models, quantitatively demonstrate how they contribute to clinical outcomes, and align with financial incentives for healthcare organizations. The pandemic has clearly demonstrated the role for laboratories and community health to support population health with consumer-driven shared decision-making models focused on improving health outcomes, reducing the overall cost of care, and decreasing prevalence of disease.

Clinical laboratories are being called to action. To achieve this vision, laboratories must take a leadership role outside of the four walls of the lab and develop key partnerships with public health and community health. Initiating these collaborations will support population health and promote both the laboratory's and community health's participation in the value-based healthcare of the future.

To support implementation, future discussions, publications, and guidance need to be developed in the following areas:

1. Identification of high priority/high yield areas of convergence for diagnostic and population health.
2. Healthcare policies and/or legislation to optimize the role of the clinical laboratory.
3. Tangible deliverables for the model that support the common vision, business model, incentives and economics.
4. Information technology needs to support data analytics and interoperability.
5. Curriculum on knowledge and management skills needed in the future clinical laboratory workforce.
6. Identification of new roles for managers and leaders in diagnostic and population health.

References:

1) Crossey M, Dodd M, VanNess R, Shotorboni, K. The lab in the time of COVID. *JALM.* 2020;5(6):1406-1407. https://doi.org/10.1093/jalm/jfaa122.

2) Kindig D, Stoddart G. What is population health? *AJPH.* 2003;93(3):380-383, https://doi.org/10.2105/AJPH.93.3.380.

3) Nash, DB. The Population Health Mandate: A Broader Approach to Care Delivery. Boardroom Press. Governance Institute.com. Published February 2012. Accessed August 2022. http://populationhealthcolloquium.com/readings/Pop_Health_Mandate_NASH_2012.pdf.

4) Shotorbani KR, Swanson KM, Bailey B.Future role of the clinical lab in population health. Population Health Management. Epub ahead of print, 13 Aug 2021: http://doi.org/10.1089/pop.2021.0167.

5) Bodenheimer T, Sinsky C. From triple to quadruple aim: care of the patient requires care of the provider. Ann Fam Med. 2014;12(6):573–576. doi: 10.1370/afm.1713.

6) Sikka R, Morath JM, Leape L. The Quadruple Aim: care, health, cost and meaning in work. BMJ Qual Saf. 2015;24:608–610.

7) Crawford JM, Shotorbani K, Sharma G, Crossey M, Kothari T, Lorey TS, et al. Improving American healthcare through "Clinical Lab 2.0." Acad Pathol. 2017:https://doi.org/10.1177/2374289517701067

8) Swanson K, Dodd M, VanNess R, Crossey M. Improving the delivery of healthcare through clinical diagnostic insights: a valuation of laboratory medicine through "Clinical Lab 2.0". J Appl Lab Med. 2018;3:487–497.

9) Shotorbani K, Orr J, Landsman K. Priming the clinical laboratory for population health. *The Pathologist.* Published 13 May 2020. Accessed August 2022. https://thepathologist.com/inside-the-lab/priming-the-clinical-laboratory-for-population-health.

10) VanNess R, Swanson K, Robertson V, Koenig M, Crossey M. The value of laboratory information augmenting a managed care organization's comprehensive diabetes care efforts in New Mexico. *JALM.* 2020;5(5):978-86. https://doi.org/10.1093/jalm/jfaa118.

11) Borunda Duque T, Dodd M, Mwithi A, VanNess R, Swanson K. Opportunity for real-time, longitudinal clinical laboratory data to enhance diabetes disease surveillance: a cross-sectional, laboratory database–enabled population study. *JALM.*2020; 5(5):967-977. https://doi.org/10.1093/jalm/jfaa106.

12) Warrington JS, Lovejoy N, Brandon J, Lavoie K, Powell C. Integrating social determinants of health and laboratory data: a pilot study to evaluate co-use of opioids and benzodiazepines. *Acad Pathol.* 2019 Jan-Dec;6:2374289519884877. Published 30 October 2019 Oct 30. Accessed August 2022.

13) Centers for Disease Control and Prevention. 10 Essential
Public Health Services. Published 9 September 2020.
Accessed August 2022.
https://www.cdc.gov/publichealthgateway/
publichealthservices/essentialhealthservices.htm

It's Not a Flip of the Switch: Piloting Screening for Social Needs in Primary Care

Brisa Urquieta de Hernandez, PhD
Holly Dockery, BS
Iris Cheng MD, FACP
Maria Reese, MPH
Alisahah Jackson, MD

AS WE RESPOND to the mounting evidence that health is determined by behavioral, socioeconomic, and environmental factors along with clinical care rather than by clinical care alone, healthcare systems have begun to shift their strategies to include addressing social risk and unmet social needs as a comprehensive way to care for patients and improve health outcomes. This practice has led to clinical care management of complex populations that includes social care integrated with medical care and broader institutional multi-sector community collaborations to address social needs. By understanding not only the clinical issues but also the social and contextual factors that impact health, providers can deliver individualized care to the whole person. While it is not expected that the healthcare provider solves, for example, food insecurity, if clinical and social systems are integrated in both data and service, a referral for fresh food should be as automatic as a primary care referral to a specialist. Can it be done? Should it be done? We will share some key findings in our research to help you connect the dots between medicine and social care interventions.

> **. . . if clinical and social systems are integrated in both data and service, a referral for fresh food should be as automatic as a primary care referral to a specialist.**

Why is Screening for Social Needs Important?

The overall health of a patient is impacted by factors that occur outside of the healthcare system: 40% of an individual's health can be attributed to socioeconomic factors, 30% to health behaviors, and 10% to physical environment. Clinical care is only responsible for 20% of a person's health status [1]. Acknowledging this evidence, health systems have begun to create strategies to address health-related social needs through intentional efforts to better understand the community level indicators impacting the health outcomes of their patients. Prior to the COVID-19 pandemic, screening for social determinants of health (SDoH) was being implemented during the clinical health assessment so that social and economic needs could be addressed [2]. Since the pandemic began, the urgency to formalize and integrate this type of screening into the clinical encounter has only increased.

In 2015, a large, integrated healthcare system in the Southeast began the process of better understanding the community and addressing its most pressing needs through convening operational leaders and subject matter experts in a workgroup to support the development of its first community health strategy [3]. Along with this, the healthcare system implemented a shift from the traditional community health needs assessments [4] required for nonprofit hospitals (since this system was a quasi-governmental healthcare system, they were exempt from this federal requirement) to an approach focused on understanding the needs of the communities served beyond a clinical lens. Believing in the power of this community-centered approach, this healthcare system developed its first strategic and comprehensive Community Health Improvement Study (CHIS) in 2016 with an intentional focus on the SDoH.

The purpose of the CHIS was to further examine the health and SDoH in all seven markets of the region to help inform the focus areas of the community health and outreach teams. The CHIS followed the eight-step process developed by the Health Research and Educational Trust: Community Health Assessment and Implementation Pathway that engages community members, local health departments, and patients in assessing population health [5]. The healthcare system collected qualitative and quantitative data, including patient data, county health rankings, focus groups, and public health reports. They collaborated with The North Carolina Institute for Public Health for data collection and analysis. This institute collected and mapped census tract-level data sourced from the US Census Bureau American Community Survey and US Department of Agriculture for twelve SDoH indicators. The twelve indicators fell within three domains: Social & Neighborhood, Economic, and Housing & Transportation. For each indicator, data was mapped using an ESRI Geographic Information System (GIS) Story Map software. Through analysis of the data, a Z score was created for each census tract displaying the highest disparities or hot spots for SDoH in an interactive story map [6].

All of this data was compiled and presented to facility and hospital leaders so they could review the information and rank the SDoH indicators based on 5 factors: magnitude, severity, urgency, vulnerable population, and interconnectedness. As a result, access to food was identified as the number one SDoH priority for the healthcare system. This report also identified the need to screen patients for social needs and link patients to social support services when appropriate.

As the health system was preparing to implement its community health strategy, the North Carolina Department of Health and Human Services (NCDHHS) was also beginning to develop strategies to address social needs to support Medicaid beneficiaries. Various state-wide workgroups were initiated to begin exploring this process. One of the groups was tasked with the development of a screening tool that would be integrated as part of Medicaid Transformation, which would require that participants of the prepaid health plans be screened for unmet social needs [7,8].

Nationally, community health centers have led the US healthcare industry with their development of various screening tools and protocols, including the PRAPARE tool (Protocol for Responding to and Assessing Patients' Assets, Risks, and Experiences). While implementation of screening has been studied in community health centers [9-11], few large healthcare systems have endeavored to systematically screen their patients for a comprehensive set of social issues across varied primary care practices [12-14]. Scaling outpatient social needs screening to adapt to the needs and resources of a large healthcare system remains a significant and largely unaddressed challenge.

> ... few large healthcare systems have endeavored to systematically screen their patients for a comprehensive set of social issues across varied primary care practices ...

As part of the screening strategy, the community health steering committee for this health system determined that it would be critical to implement small-scale pilot studies of social needs screening and evaluate these screening processes within its various ambulatory clinical environments. The goal was to identify feasible and effective processes for identifying and responding to social needs in several unique outpatient primary care settings within the healthcare system.

Pilot Process

Due to the complex nature of large healthcare systems and iterative process improvement, an opportunity to engage diverse stakeholders in the development of new workflows is not always possible. Extensive evaluation of any clinical workflow such as the screening of social needs prior to full scale implementation is necessary to better understand the barriers and facilitators to implementation. Not only does adding another process to the clinical workflow seem overwhelming to the clinical staff, but it adds a new dynamic to the interaction between the patient and the care team. Therefore, health systems need to be prepared to understand how best to integrate processes before widespread adoption of new workflows that involve the clinical staff and care teams.

Early on, we recognized that the success of the community health strategy was dependent on the collaboration of stakeholders from across health system departments and professional roles. One of the community health committees was responsible for better understanding the social and economic factors impacting patients' health. This large multidisciplinary group included participants from social work, community health work, medicine, nursing, nutrition, administration, informatics, behavioral health, research, and real estate. This committee supported two prioritized work streams: the first focused on developing interventions to address food insecurity, and the second focused on screening for social needs in the clinical settings. This group included physician champions who led and helped execute a screening pilot at their respective clinics. Engaging the care team in the development of the pilot and informing development of the screening tool was important in order to achieve early buy-in regarding this new workflow.

Seven outpatient primary care clinics (five Family Medicine, one Internal Medicine, and one Pediatrics) in urban and rural settings implemented week-long pilot studies of social needs screening. Clinic leaders, including clinicians, nurses, social workers, and administrators, designed their own process for screening implementation, with guidance from the evaluation team. At each clinic, two to four providers screened their English-speaking patients on selected days. At Family Medicine clinics, children were not screened.

A subcommittee was formed to serve as the evaluation team, and this multidisciplinary group included a health geographer, pediatrician, health policy intern, and social worker. The group developed tools that were informed by two implementation science frameworks: Consolidated Framework for Implementation Science (CFIR) and Proctor's Implementation Outcomes (Proctor) [15, 16]. Implementing a rigorous process was important to the committee because it was seen as a way to have stronger information to share when discussing scaling the screening tool. The evaluation team collected qualitative observational data during the pilot, and one member of the group completed semi-structured interviews with selected pilot participants after pilot completion.

The screening tool contained questions from two existing screening tools: the Hunger Vital Signs, developed by the US Department of Agriculture, and a subset of questions from the PRAPARE tool, developed by the National Association of Community Health Centers [11]. These questions aligned with screening domains proposed by NCDHHS [7]. The screening tool was then integrated into the healthcare system's electronic medical record (EMR) [17].

Results of the Pilots

The seven clinics adopted varying processes for social needs screening (Table 1). Allowing the clinics to inform their own process was important; although every effort is made to standardize processes and procedures across care sites, each clinical care environment inevitably becomes its own microcosm. Honoring the workflows and processes developed locally allows shared process development and supports the care team and staff to feel more comfortable integrating this new process into their workflow.

Table 1: Processes for Screening for Social Needs in Seven Outpatient Primary Care clinics

Process	FM1 (2 processes) (Urban)		FM2 (Urban)	FM3 (Rural)	FM4 (Rural)	FM5 (Urban)	IM1 (Urban)	P1 (Urban)
Introduce screener	Nurse	Provider	Registration	Nurse	Provider	Registration	Registration	Registration
Screener administration	Paper	Verbally, using EMR	On paper	On paper	On paper	On paper	On paper	On paper
Collect screener	Nurse	N/A	Nurse	Nurse	Provider	Nurse	Nurse	Nurse
Score and discuss screener	Provider	Provider	Provider	Provider	Provider	Provider	Provider	Provider
Connect to resources	Social worker	Social worker	Social worker or online resource hub	Provider via list of resources	Provider via list of resources	Social worker	Social worker	Social worker
Enter responses into EMR	Evaluator	Provider	Evaluator	Evaluator	Provider	Nurse	Provider	Evaluator

Screening rates overall were moderate, ranging from 40% to 81% of the patients who completed their appointments. The majority of patients completed the screening tool at five sites. Patients reported moderate to high rates of social needs, but few were referred to a social worker or directly to a resource (Table 2). The prevalence of social issues also varied by clinic, with the most common being food insecurity and financial strain (Table 3).

Table 2: Rates of Screening, Detection of Social Issues, and Referrals to Resources at Seven Outpatient Primary Care Clinics

Clinic	Visits (Show Rate)	Completed Screening Tool	Positive Screen	Referral Made
Family Medicine 1 (urban)	39 (80%)	31 (79%)	10 (32%)	5 (16%)
Family Medicine 2 (urban)	40 (82%)	31 (78%)	14 (45%)	8 (57%)
Pediatrics 1 (urban)	23 (79%)	14 (61%)	3 (21%)	1 (33%)
Internal Medicine 1 (urban)	37 (67%)	30 (81%)	18 (60%)	7 (39%)
Family Medicine 3 (rural)	62 (95%)	25 (40%)	8 (32%)	2 (25%)
Family Medicine 4 (rural)	58 (88%)	35 (60%)	15 (43%)	3 (20%)
Family Medicine 5 (urban)	35 (85%)	15 (43%)	10 (67%)	3 (30%)

Table 3: Prevalence of Social Issues, as Detected Through Social Needs Screening at Seven Outpatient Primary Care Clinics

Clinic	Completed Screening Tool	Identified Social Issues				
		Food Insecurity	Housing Instability	Financial Strain	Lack of Transportation	Physically or Emotionally Unsafe
FM1 (u)	31	6 (19%)	3 (10%)	4 (13%)	3 (10%)	0 (0%)
FM2 (u)	31	10 (32%)	3 (10%)	9 (29%)	6 (19%)	1 (3%)
P1 (u)	14	1 (7%)	1 (7%)	3 (21%)	1 (7%)	0 (0%)
IM1 (u)	30	13 (43%)	8 (27%)	5 (17%)	9 (30%)	4 (13%)
FM3 (r)	25	6 (24%)	3 (12%)	1 (4%)	2 (8%)	1 (4%)
FM4 (r)	35	11 (31%)	4 (11%)	10 (29%)	3 (9%)	2 (6%)
FM5 (u)	15	7 (47%)	4 (27%)	6 (40%)	2 (13%)	0 (0%)

FM = Family Medicine. P = Pediatric. IM = Internal Medicine.

After collecting observational data and completing key informant interviews using implementation science frameworks, the qualitative data was analyzed using the CFIR and Proctor framework metrics. Examples of each metric were categorized as facilitators of successful social needs screening, barriers to successful social needs screening, or neutral. Key informant interviews identified examples of these metrics and strategies to address facilitators or barriers when implementing social needs screening across the healthcare system (Table 4).

Table 4: Facilitators of and Barriers to Screening Implementation at Pilot Sites Inform the Development of a System-wide Screening Recommendation

Metric	How did it affect implementation at the pilot sites?	Impact on recommendation for system-wide strategy
FACILITATORS		
Adaptability	Clinic teams designed their own screening workflow	Allow for flexibility at clinic level and adjustment for medical specialty
Compatibility	Similar to other screening processes	Align SDOH screening with established workflows (e.g., PHQ-9 screening)
Executing	Clinics were able to execute the pilot according to plan	Processes used in the pilot can be implemented in other clinics
Goals and Feedback	Care teams understood goals of screening	Educate providers and staff on goals of screening and resource referrals
Self-Efficacy	Providers believe that they can screen for SDOH and positively impact patients	Identify provider champions to lead implementation at other clinics
Acceptability	Most patients felt comfortable answering screening questions	Add language about purpose of screening on screening form
Feasibility	Processes were carried out without outside support	Processes used in the pilot can be implemented in other clinics
BARRIERS		
Available Resources	Limited time and staff to screen and make resource referrals; Limited community resources available	Shorten screening tool to decrease time required; Increase access to social workers, community health workers, or others to provide resource referrals
Complexity	Social needs screening is a complex process, requiring coordination of multiple steps and team members	Involve multiple members of care team to minimize individual burden; Improve integration of workflow into EMR

Metric	How did it affect implementation at the pilot sites?	Impact on recommendation for system-wide strategy
Networks and Communications	Members of the care team may lack knowledge about SDOH screening, and the empathy required to screen; Social workers feel an expectation to work beyond available resources	Educate providers and staff system-wide on importance of SDOH and purpose of screening; Educate providers, staff, and patients on expectations and goals of referrals to social workers or resources
Penetration	Non-English-speaking patients not screened; Patients with low literacy not screened; Some patients not receptive to sharing personal information	Translate screening tool; Shorten screening tool to improve literacy; Decrease reading level of questions; Educate patients on importance of SDOH
Sustainability	Not feasible or appropriate to screen every patient at every visit; Cannot guarantee resource referrals when community resources are limited	Screen yearly, at a minimum, with follow-up as appropriate; Screen at continuity or wellness visits, hospital follow-up visits when possible; Educate providers, staff, and patients on expectations and goals of referrals to social workers or resources; Use data on social needs prevalence to advocate for needed services, internally and externally

What Did We Learn?

We observed a high rate of screening completion which indicates successful implementation of this screening process. However, in some clinics, there were challenges. For example, at clinic Pediatric 1, providers observed that some parents and caregivers chose not to complete the screening tool because they feared being reported to the Department of Social Services. Clinic Family Medicine 3 saw a low screening rate due to miscommunication among staff and lack of buy-in from resident physicians, as well as many patients with acute issues who did not prioritize completing the screening tool. At clinic Family Medicine 4, providers completed all aspects of the screening process themselves, from introduction of the screening tool to resource connections. These providers found this process challenging and time consuming and thus did not screen each patient. Finally, clinic Family Medicine 5 had a large Spanish-speaking population that could not complete the form which was conveyed in English.

Patients reported high rates of social needs, which suggests that screening for SDoH is appropriate and has potential to lead to addressing these patient needs and connecting patients to community resources. Echoing the findings of previous studies [6,9,14], providers and social workers expressed concerns about screening for social domains for which few or no resources are available. However, providers also indicated that regardless of resource availability, social needs screening provided valuable information that helped them to create a more appropriate care plan for the patient. This supports previous findings that social needs screening helped primary care providers know their patients better and adapt the care they provided so their clinical decisions were socially informed [13]. Additionally, data measuring the prevalence of social needs may incentivize healthcare systems to address health-related social needs and directly invest in community resources.

> ... data measuring the prevalence of social needs may incentivize healthcare systems to address health-related social needs and directly invest in community resources.

A minority of patients opted to be referred to a social worker or directly to a community resource. Low referral rates following screening have been observed in other settings [12,13,18,19]. This indicates that social needs screening is feasible, insofar as it does not overwhelm social workers' capabilities and clinic workflow. However, it may suggest the need to educate patients and clinical teams about the purpose and potential benefit of screening for social needs which can ultimately improve health outcomes. For instance, improving housing stability and food insecurity might help a patient improve how they control their diabetes. Also, there may be a lack of awareness of the availability and potential impact of community resources. The low referral rate could also be a result of the stigmatization of poverty. Importantly, it may indicate a disconnect between how healthcare systems and patients understand "need;" many patients who declined resources had normalized their experience of social need and demonstrated resilience in addressing these needs prior to screening. Healthcare systems should be mindful to respond to patients' understanding of their needs and resources rather than imposing an assumed definition of "need."

Key informants indicated that a screening process would need to align with established clinic workflows while allowing for flexibility at the individual clinic level. This desire aligns with previous research on providers' perceptions of social needs screening [10,20,21]. Based on the evaluation findings, the evaluation team developed a suggested process for social needs screening across the healthcare system's outpatient clinics:

Figure 1: Screening Workflow

Process (once per year, at continuity/wellness visit/hospital follow-up)

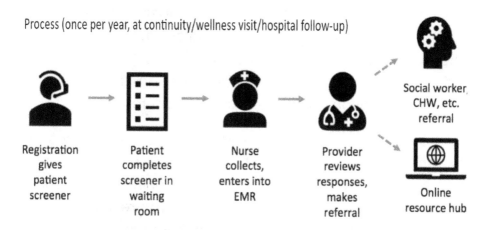

| Registration gives patient screener | Patient completes screener in waiting room | Nurse collects, enters into EMR | Provider reviews responses, makes referral | Social worker, CHW, etc. referral / Online resource hub |

(1) Registration provides the patient with the screening tool upon check-in.

(2) The patient completes the screening tool in the waiting room.

(3) The tool is given to staff rooming the patient for entry into the EMR.

(4) The provider reviews the responses listed on the screening tool by the patient.

(5) The patient and provider have a conversation about any needs.

(6) The provider makes a referral to a social worker or directly to a community resource using an online platform, as appropriate. (Figure 1)

This process shares screening tasks across multiple members of the care team, to minimize the time burden on any individual, and ensures that team members are maximizing their skill sets. The suggested clinic flow overview was informed by the seven clinics we studied but allowed for individual clinics to adjust the process to their individual patient population, clinic resources, and preferences.

The evaluation process also identified several necessary system-level changes for sustainable social needs screening in the outpatient setting. First, the screening tool must be translated into multiple languages, and the reading level of the tool should be lowered to improve accessibility, preferably to a 5th grade level. A shorter screening tool rather than the 21-item tool in our study should be developed, asking only the most relevant questions. Integration of the screening tool into the EMR should be improved, for example, by adding a biannual (or more frequent) alert in the Health Maintenance section. Given the novel aspects of addressing social needs in the clinical setting, the process for resource referrals should be strengthened by expanding the workforce and increasing access to dedicated social care personnel (social workers, community health workers, etc.) with expertise on resource navigation and social support. Questions about the patients' previous efforts to address their needs should be added to the tool to prevent repetition between primary care and social work encounters, as well as reinforce principles of empowerment and self-determination. Finally, the healthcare system should educate providers, staff members, and patients about the importance of addressing SDoH in the clinical setting, reinforcing the evidence that sharing information about social needs and connecting patients to community resources can lead to improved health outcomes [22-27].

Small-scale pilots have been successfully used to introduce SDoH screening in various settings [9,12]. This pilot was unique in that providers and clinic staff developed their own strategies for screening, and this process was evaluated using two implementation science frameworks. While the process developed in this large healthcare system may not meet the needs of every healthcare system, our lessons learned suggest that a pilot study led by providers and staff followed by a rigorous implementation evaluation is a promising strategy to inform social needs screening across a wide variety of clinic settings.

A Patient Screens Positive, Then What?

As mentioned, some of the clinics had processes suggested to allow for a direct referral to a service for the social needs that were identified while others did not. In one of the urban clinics, a process was set up for a patient who reported being food insecure to be immediately referred to an in-clinic food pharmacy for a 2-day supply of shelf stable food [28]. The patients would also have an opportunity to connect with the in-house social worker and discuss long-term solutions, including referrals to local food banks and application for Supplemental Nutrition Assistance Program (SNAP). The care team recognized that the patient is likely not the sole person in the household; therefore, additional food resources were provided that would address the needs of others in their household. It is critically important that as health systems set up processes to understand patients' needs, they also develop processes and resources to provide assistance to the patients. To this end, there are a number of social needs resource platforms that are available. As this pilot was taking place, this healthcare system was also implementing an electronic referral process utilizing the FindHelp.org (previously Aunt Bertha) platform. The care team expressed the importance of coordinating resources and documenting closed-loop referrals. Regardless of the specifics of the processes, the success of the process relies on ensuring key stakeholders are engaged and a part of the process of the conversation.

Why is This Important?

Our evaluation demonstrates that screening for SDoH was feasible in the outpatient primary care setting of a large, integrated healthcare system. However, several challenges must be addressed to ensure successful implementation, including an accessible and actionable screening tool, improved EMR integration, patient-centered timing of screening, improved resource referrals, and a widespread empathetic inquiry education to medical staff and patients about the utility of screening for social needs. Our small-scale pilot project with implementation evaluation was important in informing and preparing the healthcare system to implement social needs screenings. It was also key to supporting the care team in understanding the additional dynamic of having this type of information introduced into the patient-clinician relationship.

One family medicine physician shared the following story:

> *Patient/Person Highlight: I have been seeing a patient for almost 15 years and we never talked about any of these issues. In fact, I assumed that everything was fine since she had a full- time job with the City of Charlotte. But after she completed the screening survey, I found out she was food insecure. When I asked her about it, she said that sometimes that happens throughout the year. Now I have to think about her care differently, because she has diabetes and she may not have access to the kind of food she needs. She never shared and I never thought to ask.*

Additionally, as health systems implement community health strategies across their footprint, it is imperative to ensure engagement with both internal and external key stakeholders, particularly when it comes to screening patients for social needs. Screening for the sake of merely generating data is not the answer to addressing complex issues of health and social inequity. As these efforts continue to be implemented, it is critical to have the partnerships and resources available and accessible to support patients with unmet social needs. This is especially prudent as federal and state efforts to transform Medicaid and integrate addressing social needs are rapidly occurring. Large healthcare systems need to ensure that they themselves are serving as good partners to the organizations to which they refer their patients to address social needs. Aligning health system data and community-level data is essential to supporting the broader health of all communities served.

Key Themes:

- It is important for healthcare systems to develop their own process of implementation, engage key clinical stakeholders, and customize the pilot so that everything works for the individual clinical area.

- Healthcare teams must understand SDoH, the purpose of social needs screening, and the impact of these determinants on the health of their patients.

- Healthcare leadership must support their teams in an empathic approach to understanding social needs and adjusting and contextualizing clinical plans in order to optimize care.

- Healthcare systems must cultivate collaborative relationships with key community stakeholders who will be assisting to address social needs (food, housing, transportation, etc.)

- Healthcare systems must direct resources to address social needs as an important step to improve the health and well-being of patients with social risk. Data on social risk should not be collected simply to describe a patient population without effectively addressing these social needs.

References

1) County Health Rankings. County Health Rankings Model. http://www.countyhealthrankings.org/explore-health-rankings/measures-data-sources/county-health-rankings-model. Published 2014. Accessed May 23, 2019.

2) Gottlieb L, Sandel M, Adler NE. Collecting and applying data on social determinants of health in health care settings. JAMA Intern Med. 2013;173(11):1017-1020. doi:10.1001/jamainternmed.2013.560

3) Cheng I, Urquieta de Hernandez B, Cole A. Be the bridge. Poster presented at: Association for Community Health Improvement National Conference; April, 2017; Atlanta, GA.

4) https://www.cdc.gov/publichealthgateway/cha/plan.html.

5) Health Research &Education Trust. Engaging patients and communities in the Community Health Needs Assessment process. http://www.hpoe.org/resources/hpoehretaha-guides/2846. Published 2016. Accessed June 23, 2022.

6) Matthews GW, Cole AJ, Simon M C, Decosimo K. GIS mapping of Social Determinants of Health as a tool to facilitate community collaborations. Presentation presented at: Annual State Health Director's Conference; January 19, 2017; Raleigh, NC. Slides available at: https://doi.org/10.17615/cmge-y279.

7) North Carolina Department of Health and Human Services. Using standardized social determinants of health screening questions to identify and assist patients with unmet health-related resource needs in North Carolina. https://files.nc.gov/ncdhhs/documents/SDoH-Screening-Tool_Paper_FINAL_20180405.pdf. Published April 5, 2018. Accessed May 23, 2019.

8) Manatt Advisory Panel for the North Carolina Healthy Opportunities Pilot Service Fee Schedule. December 2018 https://www.manatt.com/commonwealthfund/healthy-opportunities-fee-schedule-advisory-panel#collapseOne_13520_1

9) Byhoff E, Cohen AJ, Hamati MC, Tatko J, Davis MM, Tipirneni R. Screening for Social Determinants of Health in Michigan health centers. J Am Board Fam Med. 2017;30(4):418-427. doi:10.3122/jabfm.2017.04.170079.

10) Byhoff E, Garg A, Pellicer M, et al. Provider and staff feedback on screening for Social and Behavioral Determinants of Health for pediatric patients. J Am Board Fam Med. 2019;32(3):297-306. doi:10.3122/jabfm.2019.03.180276.

11) National Association of Community Health Centers. PRAPARE implementation and action toolkit. http://www.nachc.org/research-and-data/prapare/toolkit/. Published 2019. Accessed May 23, 2019.

12) Buitron de la Vega P, Losi S, Sprague Martinez L, et al. Implementing an EHR-based screening and referral system

13) to address Social Determinants of Health in primary care. Med Care. 2019;57:S133-S139. doi:10.1097/MLR.0000000000001029.

14) Tong ST, Liaw WR, Kashiri PL, et al. Clinician experiences with screening for social needs in primary care. J Am Board Fam Med. 2018;31(3):351-363. doi:10.3122/jabfm.2018.03.170419.

15) Page-Reeves J, Kaufman W, Bleecker M, et al. Addressing Social Determinants of Health in a clinic setting: The WellRx Pilot in Albuquerque, New Mexico. J Am Board Fam Med. 2016;29(3):414-418. doi:10.3122/jabfm.2016.03.150272.

16) Damschroder LJ, Aron DC, Keith RE, Kirsh SR, Alexander JA, Lowery JC. Fostering implementation of health services research findings into practice: a consolidated framework for advancing implementation science. Implement Sci. 2009;4(1):50. doi:10.1186/1748-5908-4-50.

17) Proctor E, Silmere H, Raghavan R, et al. Outcomes for implementation research: Conceptual distinctions, measurement challenges, and research agenda. Adm Policy Ment Heal Ment Heal Serv Res. 2011;38(2):65-76. doi:10.1007/s10488-010-0319-7.

18) Adler NE, Stead WW. Patients in context—EHR capture of Social and Behavioral Determinants of Health. N Engl J Med. 2015;372(8):698-701. doi:10.1056/NEJMp1413945.

19) Schickedanz A, Hamity C, Rogers A, Sharp AL, Jackson A. Clinician experiences and attitudes regarding screening for Social Determinants of Health in a large integrated health system. Med Care. 2019;57:S197-S201. doi:10.1097/MLR.0000000000001051.

20) Swavely D, Whyte V, Steiner JF, Freeman SL. Complexities of addressing food insecurity in an urban population. Popul Health Manag. 2019;22(4):pop.2018.0126. doi:10.1089/pop.2018.0126.

21) Thomas-Henkel C, Schulman M. Screening for Social Determinants of Health in populations with complex needs: Implementation considerations. www.chcs.org/sdoh-screening/. Published October, 2017. Accessed May 23, 2019.

22) LaForge K, Gold R, Cottrell E, et al. How 6 organizations developed tools and processes for Social Determinants of Health screening in primary care: An overview. J Ambul Care Manage. 2018;41(1):2-14. doi:10.1097/JAC.0000000000000221.

23) Williams DR, Costa MV, Odunlami AO, Mohammed SA. Moving upstream: how interventions that address the social determinants of health can improve health and reduce disparities. Journal of Public Health Management and Practice. 2008;14(Suppl):S8.

24) Anderson KO, Green CR, Payne R. Racial and ethnic disparities in pain: causes and consequences of unequal care. The Journal of Pain. 2009;10(12),1187-1204.

25) Dzau VJ, McClellan MB, McGinnis JM, et al. Vital directions for health and health care: priorities from a National Academy of Medicine initiative. JAMA. 2017;317(14):1461-1470.

26) Daniel H, Bornstein SS, Kane GC, Health and Public Policy Committee of the American College of Physicians. Addressing social determinants to improve patient care and promote health equity: an American College of Physicians position paper. Annals of Internal Medicine. 2018;168(8):577-578

27) Artiga S, Hinton E. Beyond health care: the role of social determinants in promoting health and health equity. Health. 2019;20(10):1-13.

28) Gurewich D, Garg A, Kressin NR. Addressing social determinants of health within healthcare delivery systems: a framework to ground and inform health outcomes. Journal of General Internal Medicine, 2020;35(5):1571-1575.

29) Cooper E, Mohanan S, Garcia C, et al. An in-clinic food pharmacy addresses very low food security. Annals of Family Medicine. 2020;18(6):564-565.

Intersection Between Medicine, Physical and Mental Wellbeing, and Public Health

Meghna Patel, MHA

IMAGINE A PLACE where you could easily confirm an appointment to get an overall wellbeing check. What would that look like? It could be that you genuinely need a simple dental check-up at the moment, but you can also seamlessly get screened for physical and mental health. While getting those checkups, you also get asked if you have the proper means to live, work, eat, sleep, and enjoy life. And if you answer those questions by saying you do not have sufficient and satisfactory means, you will get quick counseling and support on the same day. Wouldn't that feel safe and empowering? Hold on to that image—we will return to this utopia at the end of the chapter.

The COVID-19 pandemic brought one silver lining: it drastically increased general awareness of mental health. Many terms have been used in this widespread awareness, such as mental health, mental illness, mental healthcare, and mental wellbeing. They may all come across as the same thing, but they actually have different definitions. According to the World Health Organization (WHO), mental health is a state of mental wellbeing that enables people to cope with the stresses of life, realize their abilities, learn well and work well, and contribute to their community. It is an integral component of health and wellbeing that underpins our individual and collective abilities to make decisions, build relationships, and shape the world we live in. Mental health is a basic human right. According to the National Alliance on Mental Illness (NAMI), mental illness is a condition that affects a person's thinking, feeling, behavior, or mood. These conditions deeply impact day-to-day living and may affect the ability to relate to others. There are two broad categories of mental illness: Any Mental Illness (AMI), where individuals may have none to mild, moderate, and even severe impairment, and Serious Mental Illness (SMI), which is a serious functional impairment that interferes with day-to-day life activities [1]. The American Psychological Association defines mental healthcare as a category of healthcare service and delivery provided by several fields involved in psychological assessment and intervention (psychology, psychiatry, neurology, social work, etc.). This type of care includes but is not limited to psychological screening and testing, psychotherapy and family therapy, and neuropsychological rehabilitation.

The COVID-19 pandemic brought one silver lining: it drastically increased general awareness of mental health.

There is no doubt mental health has an impact on physical health, and likewise, physical health has an impact on mental health. The fact is that the mind and body are not two separate entities, and one is not more significant than the other. If we look at the current state of mental health in America, suicidal ideation has drastically increased since the COVID-19 pandemic, and suicide is now one of the leading causes of death in the US. This trend is also alarming among our youth population [2]. 1 in 6 US youth aged 6-17 experience mental health disorders yearly [3].

The fact is that the mind and body are not two separate entities, and one is not more significant than the other.

Looking at the data before COVID-19, approximately 56% of patients who wanted access to a mental healthcare service faced hurdles [4]. Numerous issues prevented individuals from seeking help or being able to find a provider who accepted their insurance. There were also lengthy wait times due to shortages. Additionally, there was a general lack of awareness/screenings to assess the signs of mental illness. Finally, and, perhaps most importantly, there is stigma related to seeking mental healthcare, which has continued since the early 1800s.

Unfortunately, even with statistics this alarming, it is difficult to access care for mental health, proactively or reactively. When it comes to receiving care, why do we see hurdles? Let me ask this differently. Why do we see

Why do we see limitations in the delivery of respect for the whole body at the right time and the right place?

limitations in the delivery of respect for the whole body at the right time and the right place? Let us dive into history a bit to answer that question.

Past, Present and Hope for the Future

Back in 1908, a single person's experience and journey of getting treatment for mental illness sparked a mental hygiene movement in the US. That person's name is Clifford Beers. Beers founded the Connecticut Society for Mental Hygiene, which then became the National Committee for Mental Hygiene in 1902 and is now called Mental Health America. This movement stemmed from one of the defining objectives of public health: mental health principles should be integrated into the practices of social work, nursing, public health administration, education, industry and government [5, 6]. In 1947, The National Mental Health Act, which created the National Institute of Mental Health, passed due to Mental Health America's advocacy. However, mental health illness was still institution-led until 1963, when President Kennedy signed Community Mental Health Centers Act (CMHC), authorizing construction grants for community mental health centers. This law foundationally moved the care of individuals getting treatment for mental health from siloed institutions in the rural parts of the country to much more socially and community-supported integrated care. But did it end the practice of treating individuals with mental illness through institutions? Unfortunately, not at all. In fact, federal and state played 'pass the ball' until all the funds were drained out of the state and federal-run mental health facilities. After decades following the passage of the CMHC Act and with declining funds for outpatient centers, which, along with the increased demand for mental health services, there were increasing levels of unmet mental health needs. With limited public funding to support CMHC, agencies became increasingly reliant on managed care entities. While the emergence of managed care in the United States allowed for the survival and expansion of mental health services, in some ways, it resulted in a shift away from addressing the needs of individuals with mental health illness, many of whom were unlikely to have access to insurance or affordable coverage. One such negative impact of this was that individuals treated within their community were often unable to sustain satisfactory community participation, ultimately resulting in them being incarcerated. This journey sparked long-lasting stigma in the community, preventing the work CMHC was established to do in the first place.

Many essential laws and regulations have been achieved since then to ensure access and advocacy for individuals needing mental healthcare, such as the Protection and Advocacy for Mentally Ill Act, Americans with Disabilities Act, Children's Health Act, Garrett Lee Smith Memorial Act, Mental Health Parity and Addiction Equity Act, Affordable Care Act, Comprehensive Addiction and Recovery Act, 21st Century Cures Act, SUPPORT Act, and many other state laws and regulations. In 2022, we saw the most significant funding ($10 billion) in the history of mental health access and advocacy enacted through the Bipartisan Safer Communities Act. It is an excellent investment. COVID-19 expedited access to mental healthcare services with telehealth innovations and created more scrutiny into lack of health insurance coverages and loopholes, etc.

While there have been some advancements, there is plenty of evidence that the impact of this pandemic (ie., deaths, long COVID, political distress, etc.) combined with economic and social turmoil will ring for decades. Will all of this current investment help solve what was severely inequitable before and during the pandemic? The short answer is yes—somewhat, and this answer comes from a place of hope and from seeing positive outcomes. We will touch upon this shortly.

Our Big Hurdle

So far, all we've highlighted is just mental health. We haven't even mentioned the disease of addiction called substance-use disorder. A 2018 National Survey on Drug Use and Health highlighted that over 9.2 million adults in the US have co-occurring mental illness and substance-use disorder [7]. Before the pandemic, public health and safety responded hands-on to the rising drug-related overdose epidemic. We know the cause of overdoses, and the epidemic's trajectory shifted from prescription opioids to illicit substance use-related overdoses. In recent years, the rate of overdoses has gone up drastically because the drugs are laced with fentanyl, a dangerous synthetic opioid that is 50 times stronger than heroin. More than 107,600 lives have been lost from drug-related overdoses in 2021, the highest annual death toll on record. All these deaths are preventable. Yes, they are preventable, and, rightly so, through proper care coordination. A staggering 43% of U.S. adults who say they needed substance-use or mental healthcare in the past 12 months did not receive that care, and numerous barriers to access stand between them and needed treatment [8]. That's our big hurdle.

Indeed, COVID-19 highlighted healthcare's nightmare of addressing a pandemic amid a growing epidemic during a looming mental health crisis. It remains a nightmare for public health professionals and providers who practice medicine.

Primary Care + Public Health = Good News!

Both mental illnesses and substance-use disorders have a variety of treatment modalities—from counseling and therapies to residential and hospital-based treatment, medication-assisted treatment, telehealth, and recovery support services. The primary care framework emphasizes that patients' access to efficient, equitable, and effective primary care services should be of the highest quality leading to better care, better health, and lower costs. If we know that the primary care framework can have these outcomes, why do we continue to hear about the lack of or the importance of integrating behavioral health and primary care to improve patients' clinical outcomes? It brings us back to our original question, ie., hurdles in accessing whole person care. It may surprise you, but in many ways, primary care practices have acted as the mental healthcare providers, in some cases continuing to refer patients to social care services, but this is not always consistent across the nation. This is inconsistent due to a lack of skilled clinical and nonclinical resources, technology infrastructure, reimbursement of care models, and persistent fatigue and burnout leading to these care gaps. The primary care model is also not required to provide these services—partly because they continue to face challenges around not being considered "experts" regarding mental healthcare and social service providers.

On the other hand, public health continues to see the effects and outcomes of population health, making it even harder to address the social determinants of health because of this fragmented system. Moreover, public health authorities don't have any regulating or licensing oversight over healthcare providers in similar ways to State Licensing Boards, State Medicaid, and the Centers for Medicare and Medicaid Services. But, even in the face of these challenges, public health continues to build promotion resources and intervention tactics through evidence and research to prevent disease, both mental and physical.

The good news is that we have plenty of opportunities to align and join forces from local, state, and federal public health authorities with our healthcare providers who deliver care directly to individuals. We have solid reasons and promising results for closing this damaging gap. We have examples where this has already happened—there is a success rate—and we can all learn from and continue to bridge those gaps [9]. Two such measures in the realm of mental health illness and substance-use prevention come to mind.

Partnership + Access = Improved Outcomes

The first example is evidence of the impact of Certified Community Behavioral Health Clinics (CCBHCs). CCBHCs is a model of care funded through the Protecting Access to Medicare Act of 2014. A CCBHC model provides community-based mental health and substance-use disorder services, advancing behavioral health integration with physical healthcare by using evidence-based practices and promoting improved access to high-quality care. Care coordination is the linchpin holding these aspects of the clinic and ensuring that this is provided 24/7 to individuals who may or may not have insurance coverage. Moreover, CCBHCs must build innovative partnerships with law enforcement, social service programs, schools, and hospitals to improve overall health, reduce recidivism, and prevent hospital readmissions [10]. Remember that WHO defines mental health as a fundamental human right? This model is a starting point for the CCBHC path.

The Substance Abuse and Mental Health Services Administration (SAMHSA) leads public health efforts to advance the nation's behavioral health and improve the lives of individuals living with mental and substance-use disorders and their families. SAMHSA oversees the implementation and expansion of the CCBHC model. As of mid-2022, over 450 CCBHCs operate from 42 states and Guam. Almost every summer, the National Council for Mental Wellbeing prepares an impact report around critical findings from the CCBHC model. These findings have shown that states reported reductions in Emergency Department (ED) visits, reduced law enforcement involvement, and increased evidence-based services like medication-assisted treatment, reducing the total cost of care. So, for instance, 76% of patients under the supervision of this model in the state of Missouri have experienced reduced ED visits and hospitalizations, and, in cases where these patients had involvement with law enforcement, about 70% had no further involvement within six months. Multiple states, including Minnesota, Missouri, New Jersey, Nevada, and Oregon, reported that the CCBHC model led to a significant expansion of peer workers and family support specialists, individuals with lived experience of mental health or substance-use conditions who support coordination and understanding of services for new clients [11]. Now, this was all possible from a minimal funding investment paired with the initial payment demonstration model established by the CMS. After this model was introduced in Texas, we even saw a successful state-level agency collaboration and integration of oversight and services to the public through the Texas CCBHC initiative. Essentially, the Texas Health and Human Services Commission (HHSC) was directed to re-align and consolidate functions across all HHS agencies to improve efficiency and delivery of services. As a result of this legislative direction, in September 2016, the State's public health, mental health, and substance abuse authority's (MHSA) function of the Texas Department of State Health Services (DSHS) became part of HHSC, consolidating all community-based behavioral health functions within one [12].

Because of this continued impact of the model, the Bipartisan Safer Communities Act committed over $10 billion that will be establishing these clinics around the country. Remember how we questioned the investment?

> **Through evidence and sustainability, integrated care shows positive population outcomes—a ray of hope in whole person care.**

This investment is how we will continue to close the fragmented and inequitable care gap! Through evidence and sustainability, integrated care shows positive population outcomes—a ray of hope in whole person care.

Evidence Based Data in Action

Another example is the State Prescription Drug Monitoring Programs (PDMPs) that continue to present evidence-based public health, clinical practice, and a health IT tool. This program ensures that patients are protected from any risks of overprescribing and overlapping dangerous combinations of medications leading to overdoses. Historically, PDMPs have been around in the US since the early 1940s and have always remained a law enforcement tool. Still, since early 2016, they have presented a promising tool for healthcare providers in curbing the opioid epidemic. As a clinical tool, providers can see their own prescribing trends, sometimes compared to other providers in their specialty group, and receive proactive alerts when there seems to be a close call towards a dangerous threshold of prescribing to a patient. Timely data, like in a "real-time" PDMP, maximizes the utility of the prescription history data, with significant implications for patient safety and public health. Some may argue that the pendulum swung too far to the other side when PDMP use was mandated for providers. Of course, the public health departments did observe that patients were dropped from care due to suspicious doctor shopping activities. However, public health agencies tried to curb that through proper academic detailing and education-empowered clinicians to ensure patients have access to safe, effective pain management while also treating substance-use disorder. The Pennsylvania Department of Health (PA DOH) developed specialty-specific opioid prescribing guidelines since CDC guidelines were initially misleading [13]. To mitigate this confusion, the PA DOH developed Evidence-Based Prescribing: Tools You Can Use to Fight the Opioid Epidemic education curriculum, where training was provided on effectively using the PDMP system to make informed clinical decisions.

PA DOH also leveraged PDMP for patient advocacy, support, and referral to better treatment providers. In instances where a provider could not prescribe proper medications due to a regulatory or a law enforcement action, the Health Department would work with the patient's health insurer and other state agencies. The patient could seamlessly find another clinician to provide pain management and substance-use disorder treatment in that process [14]. Through 49 state PDMPs, evidence shows that it helped clinicians with prescribing practices and gave a clear picture of the medication history of patients undergoing severe mental health illnesses and substance-use disorders.

Enhanced Collaboration

Additionally, syndromic surveillance is another example of an enhanced collaboration between public health agencies, healthcare providers, and hospitals. In late September of 2017, Pennsylvania was the first of 16 states to receive the Enhanced State Opioid Overdose Surveillance Program grant. Before this grant funding, Pennsylvania, like many other states, could not collect rapid information on fatal and nonfatal overdoses. It was a continuous collaboration with the EDs and the connectivity with their respective electronic health records (EHRs) to receive prompt admission, discharge, and transfer data, along with a strong and sensitive partnership with Medical Examiners and

Coroners of the state. Through this collaboration, the health department collected and alerted county case workers for referral to treatment, EMS, and law enforcement of any upticks in drug overdoses in their communities.

A Healthy America: Physical & Mental Health

These examples demonstrate that a strong partnership between public health and the healthcare delivery system could bring a solid, comprehensive care experience for individuals seeking care. If two systems of care join forces to work together, they can solve preventable health challenges at the community level. The critical return on investment will always be a healthy America, one community at a time.

Early in this chapter, we asked you to imagine a place where you could get health and social care services, all in one place. After reading about these examples and the progress of the public health and healthcare delivery partnership, this feels less like an impossible utopia and more like a possible reality for everyone. Our collective drive and need for equitable access to quality care are helping to accomplish this.

Public Health 3.0, released in 2016, called for action for all traditional public health departments to enhance the current infrastructure and broaden their work by building strategic partnerships. The term "Public Health 3.0" meant to bring "modernization" of public health, was coined in 2016 by Karen B. DeSalvo, MD, MPH, MSc [15]. Fast forward to 2022, after learnings from the COVID-19 pandemic, public health should work hand in hand with other sectors of healthcare like the hospitals, health systems, community health providers, and pharmacists to forecast, prevent, intervene, and ensure a safe and healthy society for everyone.

References:

1) National Institute of Mental Health. Mental illness. Updated January 2022. Accessed August 31, 2022. https://www.nimh.nih.gov/health/statistics/mental-illness.

2) Mental Health America. The state of mental health in America. Published 2022. Accessed August 31, 2022. https://www.mhanational.org/issues/state-mental-health-america.

3) National Alliance on Mental Illness. Mental health by the numbers. Updated June 2022. Accessed August 31, 2022. https://www.nami.org/mhstats.

4) Cohen Veterans Network and the National Council for Behavioral Health. America's mental health 2018. Published October 10, 2018. Accessed August 31, 2022. https://www.cohenveteransnetwork.org/wp-content/uploads/2018/10/Research-Summary-10-10-2018.pdf.

5) Parry M. From a patient's perspective: Clifford Whittingham Beers' work to reform mental health services. *Am J Public Health*. 2010;100(12):2356-2357. doi: 10.2105/AJPH.2010.191411.

6) Mandell W. The realization of an idea. Department of Mental Health website. Johns Hopkins, Bloomberg School of Public Health. Published in 1995. Accessed September 16, 2022. https://publichealth.jhu.edu/departments/mental-health/about/origins-of-mental-health).

7) Substance Abuse and Mental Health Services
Administration. Key substance use and mental health
indicators in the United States: results from the 2019 National
Survey on Drug Use and Health. Published May 2019.
Accessed August 31, 2022.
https://store.samhsa.gov/product/key-substance-use-
and-mental-health-indicators-in-the-united-states-results-
from-the-2018-national-survey-on-Drug-Use-and-
Health/PEP19-5068.

8) National Council for Mental Wellbeing. 2022 Access to Care
survey results. Published May 31, 2022. Accessed August 31,
2022. https://www.thenationalcouncil.org/2022-access-to-
care-survey/.

9) Gaertner SJ, Krishnasamy VP, Simone PM, Schuchat A.
Leveraging rapid response activities to build public health
capacity: development of the opioid rapid response team
model. *Health Security*. 2022; 20(1): 87-91.
https://doi.org/10.1089/hs.2021.0008.

10) Substance Abuse and Mental Health Services
Administration. Criteria for the demonstration program to
improve Community Mental Health Centers and to establish
Certified Community Behavioral Health Clinics. Published
May 2016. Accessed August 31, 2022.
https://www.samhsa.gov/sites/default/files/programs_ca
mpaigns/ccbhc-criteria.pdf.

11) National Council for Mental Wellbeing. Transforming state behavioral health systems: findings from states on the impact of CCBHC implementation. Published October 2021. Accessed August 31, 2022. https://www.thenationalcouncil.org/wp-content/uploads/2022/02/Transforming-State-Behavioral-Health-Systems.pdf.

12) Texas CCBHC demonstration application. Published October 2016. Accessed August 31, 2022. https://www.hhs.texas.gov/sites/default/files/documents/doing-business-with-hhs/providers/health/ccbhc/ccbhc-demonstration-application-narrative.pdf.

13) Pennsylvania Department of Health. Opioid Prescribing Guidelines. Accessed September 16, 2022. https://www.health.pa.gov/topics/disease/Opioids/Pages/Prescribing-Guidelines.aspx.

14) Pennsylvania Department of Health. Patient advocacy program. Published December 2019. August 31, 2022._ https://www.health.pa.gov/topics/programs/Patient-Advocacy/Pages/Patient%20Advocacy.aspx.

15) DeSalvo KB, Wang YC, Harris A, Auerbach J, Koo D, O'Carroll P. Public health 3.0: A call to action for public health to meet the challenges of the 21st century. *Prev Chronic Dis.* 2017;14:170017. doi: http://dx.doi.org/10.5888/pcd14.170017.

Whole Person Index: Now I'm a Believer

Dr. Katie Kaney, DrPH, MBA, FACHE
Carolyn Minnock, MBA

IF YOU HAVE a conversation with anyone about health or healthcare, inevitably data, analytics, and artificial intelligence (AI) are discussed at some point. This trifecta has become part of the healthcare conversation because of its predictivity and power to prioritize the vast amounts of information at our collective fingertips. We are believers.

While we are believers in the power of data, analytics, and AI, we recognize that the current use of these tools perpetuates the traditional healthcare model, using data such as claims information and past utilization to predict future market share and demand. Usable data is also just beginning to be unleashed as the initial promise of interoperability may now be at a point of realization. Furthermore, consumer-driven health, while an industry favorite buzzword, has not been prioritized in the traditional sick-driven healthcare system.

Viable distribution channels and tools now ubiquitous such as telemedicine and health bots, capturing data from a different demographic of health users, position true consumer-driven healthcare as a formidable player.

The American health system is flush with best-in-class data, analytics, technology, academic prowess, and solutions. Why then, are indicators such as lifespan declining and variances in lifespan by race and gender increasing?[1]

In this chapter, we will offer some thoughts on this question. We will also offer a new approach that we believe can create balance in our system and address health by harnessing focus, transparency, outcomes measurement, continuous improvement, and accountability. This approach is built on the Whole Person Index (WPI).

Drivers of Health

The overall drivers of health include clinical (10%), social (20%), genetic (30%), and behavior (40%) [2].

Over 80% of health spending is on clinical services [3].

When you take a moment to think about the last two statements, you might have to pause. Really? Is this true? Can it be? But another question to ask is, is this information positive or

Over 80% of health spending is on clinical services.

negative? The answer may depend on your angle and position in the health equation.

The current system of health, and healthcare, produces gaps in care, creating health inequity [4]. This statement also causes most people to pause. Why does the American health system perpetuate health inequity? Let's go back to all the drivers of health and take each, one at a time:

- Clinical treatment is largely built to treat sickness, often reactively.
- Social treatment is often fragmented, less understood scientifically, and difficult to scale.
- Genetic treatment is not widely available for mainstream application.
- Behavior treatment to positively impact behavior choice is not fully integrated into the health continuum; often it is considered too difficult to change personal choice.

As you read and thought about the last few facts and statements, what picture of health did you have in your mind? Was it clinically focused—for example, involving doctors, hospitals, and/or pharmaceuticals—or did you think about viruses or environmental factors? Or behaviors such as smoking, drinking, or exercise? Or your relative who died of breast cancer or who has high blood pressure?

All of these images *are* correct. Each of the examples above are elements which drive your health. But the reality is that the sum of all factors—clinical, social, genetic, and behavior—drive your ultimate health stability.

If you reflect on your answers and then take a broader view of all health drivers—recognizing that all drivers are important—the next practical questions are as follows:

1. What do I know about my health drivers?
2. What can I do about my drivers?

An Index for Action that Combines All Health Drivers

A scan of the landscape reveals many products which consolidate data, provide benchmarking and trending, and serve it up to teams to support decision-making. Within public health, indices such as the Vulnerability Index and Community Health Needs Assessment utilize population level data and drive to a community level for implementation. In healthcare, the best practices reflected in national regulations and registries compile individual clinical information to predict demise and prioritize interventions. The focus on health equity has given rise to companies focused on the social determinants of health (SDoH), and the federal government is requiring reporting starting in 2023 to begin to consolidate data to formalize a plan to address health inequity. Precision medicine is making great strides, with increasing ability to tailor treatments or prevention measures based upon your genetic lineage and profile. The arena of behavior change is defined with success in many retail and wellness areas, prompting action by individuals and communities.

These products show that we are working in each of the four health driver areas, but most focus on a singular aspect. This does not mean that these products are not useful, but they are, however, incomplete. Each of these products aligns their effort to a single driver of health, instead of the full scope of *all* drivers of health.

Furthermore, our use of these products assumes all drivers of health are of equal importance, or that the area you have the most access to or the most attention for wins the prize for the focus. As we pointed out from the Kaiser Family Foundation research [2], driver impact is not equally distributed. The current approach is out of balance with a majority of funding (80%) aligned to clinical drivers, but these clinical drivers only contribute to 10% of health.

> ... **driver impact is not equally distributed. The current approach is out of balance ...**

This leads us to our hypothesis and the motivation for the Whole Person Index:

We hypothesize that health for individuals and populations will be improved if all drivers of health—clinical, social, genetic, and behavior—are scientifically understood and treated in a balanced approach.

- Right now, there is no scientifically valid product supporting knowledge and action around all drivers of health together—clinical, social, genetic, behavior.
- A scientifically vetted predictive analytics index that includes all drivers—a Whole Person Index—will validate the impact of all drivers, spurring change in knowledge, treatment value, payment, and practice.

- A Whole Person Index, reliably applied, will set new health outcome standards and paths to achieve.
- Scientifically valid, actionable information with practical, cost-effective solutions will catalyze incentive change.
- Incentive change will transform the health system, and the health of people and populations, as we know it.

Makes Sense, but Easier Said than Done!

As we know and is stated throughout the book, change is difficult. Very difficult. The current economic engine of health is driven by healthcare services, largely clinical treatments and solutions. The current healthcare system is built to address sickness, largely reactively. The current public health system is built to address populations, largely focused on the underserved. Both medicine and public health are not lacking data. However, data turned into meaningful information by which a person's health can be assessed from the lens of all drivers, objectively and risk stratified with sensitivity to clinical, social, genetic, and behavior predisposition is not readily available. Furthermore, it is not validated with scientific understanding of causal relationships and root cause analysis to support systemic treatments. Whew.

Can We Find a Solution? Yes! I'm a Believer. Let's Do It.

Within the clinical domain, there are options with a proven track record of providing reliable data and analytics in a usable format to address clinical changes in care to prevent demise and support physiological stability.

Post-pandemic, the application of data integration and scientific rigor applied to the SDoH is a hot topic. Many products are in-process and people are hard at work to bring these to market to address more social drivers. This is all a step in the right direction. However, creating a tool to prioritize social and not clinical drivers, or vice versa, in essence perpetuates the current problem.

If you only focus on clinical and social, you are only getting 30% of the pie. We want the whole pie.

No one is truly aware or "treating" all drivers of health— rather, they are using the tools in their tool kit without a full scope of understanding of other health factors. This is okay—it should not be assumed that physicians can solve all of the issues or that public health professionals can close all of the gaps, or that changing behaviors alone will be enough.

The power is in the integration of the expertise across all drivers—informed by data and science. The hypothesis is that providing the same focus and rigor to drive

The power is in the integration of the expertise across all drivers— informed by data and

prioritization and implementation of action to support solutions for all drivers of health is necessary.

Figure 1: Whole Person Index = Clinical + Social+Genetic + Behavior

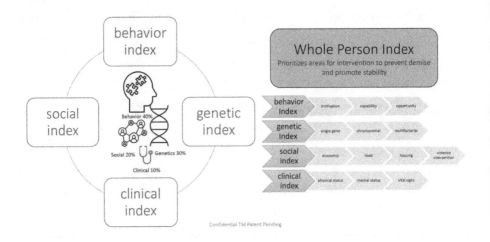

Source: Kaney

A scientifically valid predictive analytics index to include clinical, social, genetic, and behavior drivers to create a Whole Person Index (Figure 1) will be very valuable in the market. The Whole Person Index:

- Supports a comprehensive view of all health drivers—clinical (10%), social (20%), genetic (30%), and behavior (40%).
- Uses scientifically valid methodology and predictive analytics to "score" stability for each health driver, summarized by an index.
- Contains details on specific areas of opportunity to best promote stability.
- Informs prioritization, personalization, and a balanced treatment approach.

- Aligns drivers and outcomes for skill match and accountability.
- Offers reliable reporting, benchmarking, trending for outcomes management, payment, regulatory reporting, and continuous improvement.
- Provides a path to improved health outcomes at a lower cost.

Whole Person Index: Idea to Reality

While we believe it is the time for a different path to truly achieve improved health outcomes for all, we also believe that an additive approach without rigor or scientific validity would cause more challenges. From this point forward, we cannot be okay with approaching health with a focus on just one or two of the drivers. For the United States to markedly improve its current health status, the recognition of the whole, in addition to its parts and how they are inextricably linked, is mandatory.

The good news with this approach is there is very effective work being done in each of the health driver "parts."

The goal is not to duplicate. Instead, the goal is to recognize the driver experts and convene them to share their perspective and experience. By aggregation of data, analytics, and outcomes, we will apply science to understand the status of each health driver and, furthermore, how they relate to each other. The insight by individual, population, and cohort will be served up in current workflow for understanding and action.

The underpinning of a repository for continuous learning, advancement of benchmarks, trending, and outcomes management is critical to success.

Let's take an example—meet Danny:

Figure 2: Whole Person Index in Action

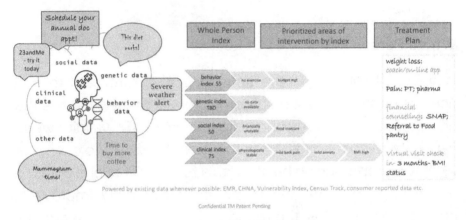

Source: Kaney

Danny is a 38-year-old female (Figure 2).

On the left you can see the input of messages in Danny's life that impact her health stability. Overlaying the data science, an index score is assigned to Danny for each health driver (100: most stable; 0 least stable).

- <u>Clinical index</u>: 75—stable—experiencing mild anxiety and a BMI that's a little too high. This could place Danny in a 'rising risk' clinical category.
- <u>Social index</u>: 50—unstable—noting the financial difficulty she is facing and further impact of the struggle to afford food.

- <u>Genetic index:</u> there is currently no data input
- <u>Behavior index:</u> 55—unstable—recently abandoning her exercise routine and facing financial issues with a car broken down and rent recently increased.

Based upon this information and engagement with Danny, the following treatment plan was "prescribed," aligning with her specific data points on her drivers of health but validated by scientifically valid analytics and AI. This includes a behavioral health specialist to discuss the anxiety, an online weight management app with coach, a financial counselor to discuss budget management and options, a referral to the local food pantry, and a virtual follow-up visit with her doctor to check in on her BMI and anxiety status.

Wow! This is a lot to digest and perhaps a lot to do. For anyone. Remember, change is hard, for most of us. But, these changes are necessary if we want to bring visibility to all drivers and achieve more positive outcomes for more people; the Whole Person Index can make these changes a little bit easier. Once we have the drivers understood, gaps identified, and solutions aligned, we provide a path to health which is more comprehensive and, in turn, more efficient and effective.

Reactive to Proactive: Individuals, Populations, and Communities

The additional piece of AI applied would be able to draw a comparison group for Danny and help to prioritize the interventions recommended for the highest likelihood to impact ratio on overall health stability. This would allow us to meet Danny as an individual, but it would also allow us to learn from populations and communities, to proactively intervene to align solutions across the drivers.

The science will be continuously refined to 'prove' the importance of all drivers and their prioritization within each and across each driver, along with the effectiveness of diversified treatments across drivers. The ability of the science and data to inform the priorities should lead to changing of incentives, payment, treatments, and ultimately achievement of better outcomes (Figure 3).

Figure 3: Whole Person Index: Individual, Population , and Community

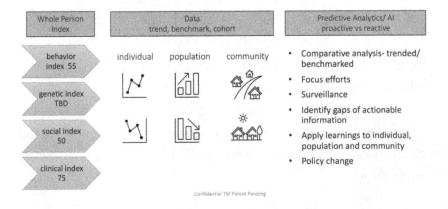

Source: Kaney

In the wise words of a surgeon who has been as much of a champion as a critic—we want to be focused on not just change but change for measurable, sustainable, scalable outcomes—

"*In the end, to shift resources to other areas, one must have a path for success which is more valuable, proven, and sustainable.*"

We believe understanding *all* drivers of health and supporting a system to effectively provide solutions across all drivers with the Whole Person Index is a path worth pursuing. We are pragmatic, at best, and frustrated with the current ineffective system, at worst. We expect ourselves, as leaders, to be part of a meaningful change to be better for all those counting on us, and this, quite simply, is the reason we are doing this work. We welcome other believers to join us today.

References:

1) Arias E, Tejada-Vera B, Kochanek K, Ahmad F. Provisional life expectancy estimates for 2021. *Vital Statistics Rapid Release*. 2022; 23; 2022. https://www.cdc.gov/nchs/data/vsrr/vsrr023.pdf

2) Artiga S, Hinto E. Beyond health care: The role of social determinants in promoting health and health equity. Kaiser Family Foundation.org. Published May 10, 2018. Accessed September 29, 2022. https://www.kff.org/racial-equity-and-health-policy/issue-brief/beyond-health-care-the-role-of-social-determinants-in-promoting-health-and-health-equity/.

3) Bipartisan Policy Center. What makes us healthy vs. what we spend on being healthy. Published June 5, 2012. Accessed September 29, 2022. https://bipartisanpolicy.org/report/what-makes-us-healthy-vs-what-we-spend-on-being-healthy/.

4) Schneider EC, Shah A, Doty MM, Tikkanen R, Fields K, Williams II RD. Mirror, Mirror, 2021: Reflecting poorly: health care in the U.S. compared to other high-income countries. The Commonwealth Fund.org. Published August 4, 2021. Accessed September 29, 2022. https://www.commonwealthfund.org/publications/fund-reports/2021/aug/mirror-mirror-2021-reflecting-poorly.

Redefining Roles—Payer

Brian Sneve, MPH

MY ROLE IN this book is to outline for you an argument for transformation. This argument is not for transformation of regulated systems, which in our fractured body politic look increasingly infeasible, but for the transformation of the relationships that drive our health system in the United States. The intent of these newfound relationships is to relegate the competitions and contentions that have defined our past to history and approach our shared problems (and opportunities) as a united front. The key to this revolution is a reimagination of the role of payers in the United States, a shift away from the perception of their role as money-doling middle people and toward a vision of payers as stewards of the value of care, partners in the creation of health, and incubators of innovation in the field of population health.

A brief explanation of terms deliberately used in this context:

> PayER—Health insurance entities designed to take the risk pool associated with a population to defray the potential costs of health costs.

> PayOR—Any individual or entity that pays the cost for healthcare expense (e.g., individuals bearing the cost of uninsurance or health insurance entities organizing risk pools).

In this context, not all Pay**ors** are Pay**ers**, but all Pay**ers** are Pay**ors**.

Opportunity—Means—Motive

Before I present the crux of my argument, I believe it is important to assess the current state of insurance in the US. There are any number of organizations that regularly report on the status of the health insurance market, probably none more commonly cited than the Kaiser Family Foundation (KFF). Citing 2019 American Community Survey (ACS) data, they report that in 2019, 50% of the population was insured by Employer Sponsored Insurance (ESI) and a further 6% were covered by individual purchased insurance from private insurers (Figure 1) [1].

Figure 1: Insurance Coverage by Type of Insurance 2019

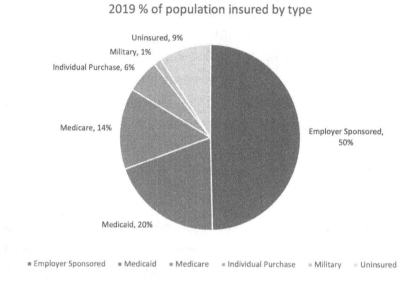

2019 % of population insured by type

Uninsured, 9%
Military, 1%
Individual Purchase, 6%
Medicare, 14%
Employer Sponsored, 50%
Medicaid, 20%

■ Employer Sponsored   ■ Medicaid   ■ Medicare   ■ Individual Purchase   ■ Military   ■ Uninsured

In separate reports during this same time period, KFF reported that 69% of Medicaid members were participating in Managed Care Organizations (MCOs)—privately managed Medicaid plans [2]—and the Department of Health and Human Services reported that 37% of Medicare enrollees were enrolled in privately underwritten Medicare Advantage plans [3]. All told, this indicates that over 68% of the population was covered by a private insurance company policy in 2019, even if the individual enrollee was subscribed to a "public" insurance option. This privatization of public insurance options is increasing: the same KFF data that supplied the 2019 Medicaid MCO enrollment numbers indicated that in 2020 enrollment in MCOs jumped to 74% [2]. In 2021, states like North Carolina joined the Managed Medicaid trend, bringing the total of states with some form of Managed Medicaid waiver to 41 [4]. Medicare Advantage continues to see similar growth trends, with KFF reporting that in 2021 42% of eligible Medicare enrollees had enrolled in a Medicare Advantage plan, up a full 11% from only 5 years before—a 35% increase over that time period [5]. The opportunity for private insurers to reach and influence the health of the population is strong and increasing.

Economically, private health insurance payers are raging juggernauts compared to the funding afforded to traditional public health organizations. In a 2022 report on the 2021 performance of insurance plans, the National Association of Insurance Commissioners (NAIC) reported that, for those health insurance plans required to report to State Commissioners of Insurance (not all states have a commissioner), Net Earned Premiums (NEP) exceeded $890 billion [6] for fully insured products. I have to highlight that this is not inclusive of the full premium gathered for private health insurance payers, merely the best single source we have for the industry—the true total is higher. This huge sum stands in stark contrast to the funding available for traditional public health efforts. A 2022 report from the Trust for America's Health reported that total funding for the Centers for Disease Control programs in 2021 was $8.26 billion and state public health funding was $14.7 billion (five states including DE, KS, RI, UT, and WV did not report public health spending) [7]. Private industry insurance payer funding exceeds public health funding (non-pandemic) by *at least 38-fold.* Private health insurers represent an ample—and largely untapped—means for funding population health efforts.

That same NAIC report indicates that the health insurance industry spent $775 billion on Medical/Pharmacy Costs [6], revealing that insurance companies spent roughly 87% of their NEP on medical costs (known as the Medical Loss Ratio or MLR). Various state and federal laws regulate the minimum MLR that a plan <u>must</u> spend or be required to repay the unmatched premiums to subscribers. This standard is set by the Patient Protection and Affordable Care Act's (PPACA) requirement that an average of 85% of premium be spent on medical costs over a three-year period for Large Group coverage and a minimum 80% MLR on Individual and Small Group products sold on the exchanges [8]. While this required MLR varies by Line of Business (LOB) and location of coverage, operating constraints and industry competition often holds the MLR to the 85% target. Based on the NAIC report, we can see that insurers have space to improve. This 2% variance from the 85% standard represents *missed margin opportunity.* In other words, although insurers are often accused of unabashedly seeking profit, they frequently do not achieve all of the potential margin that they are legally allowed to collect.

> **Taken together these facts highlight that the private health payer industry is primed (with strong means, motive, and opportunity) for an expanded role in population health improvement beyond their traditional role of claims processors and financial intermediaries.**

The positive and negative implication of this is that they are motivated to decrease the cost of care to improve their financial performance.

Taken together these facts highlight that the private health payer industry is primed (with strong means, motive, and opportunity) for an expanded role in population health improvement beyond their traditional role of claims processors and financial intermediaries.

Redefining "Value" in Healthcare

One of the issues that has kept payers from realizing this population health opportunity is an antiquated interpretation of the value proposition that health insurers provided to their enrollees. The foundations of insurance in the United States are imbedded in the Great Depression, when hospitals saw shrinking occupancy rates and rising uncompensated care. An enterprising administrator at Baylor College devised a way to provide durable revenue: for 50 cents a month, he offered up to 21 days of care in the hospital for enrollees. This plan eventually became the nation's first Blue Shield© Plan [9].

Health insurance, in particular comprehensive health insurance (provider and hospital coverage in one service) in the United States, found its footing during the second World War. Efforts to stem inflation limited employers ability to increase wages to attract limited wartime human resources, and they began to offer health insurance benefits as an incentive to employment [10]. This economic motivation simultaneously normalized what had been a relatively rare commodity and entrenched ESI as a key feature of the American health system. It also entrenched within payers a value proposition based simply on economic exchange. The general consumer of health insurance was perceived to be looking for the best coverage at the lowest price. This drove the health insurance industry to pursue more and more aggressive cost-saving measures in order to combat medical cost inflation and hold premiums at a level where consumers would be willing to pay. Concepts like "narrow networks," "Health Maintenance Organizations (HMOs),"' and "High Deductible Health Plans (HDHPs)" fell in and out of vogue—all in pursuit of an antiquated perception of what consumers valued from health insurance.

If you, the reader, will forgive the brief and extremely abridged history lesson, the remainder of this section will deal with a key aspect of transformation: the redefinition of value from the payer perspective. The topics presented were developed by the Institute for Healthcare Improvement (IHI) and intended primarily for implementation within provider systems, but, in keeping with the content of this chapter, I will argue that payers have just as much of a role in enacting the models proposed. The specific model I reference was fully described by Nundy et al. [11] in January of 2022, published in the *Journal of the American Medical Association*, and it is an expansion on the quadruple aim model that has prevailed since 2014.

The original model, initially coined the triple aim (IHI 2007) [12], sought to describe the value of healthcare as the confluence of three paradigms: 1) Patient Experience 2) Quality of Care 3) Reductions in the Cost of Care. In 2014, IHI added the fourth aim, Provider Access/Retention [11]. The quintuple aim embraces a concept that is finally getting deserved traction in healthcare and public health: Health Equity. The concept, outlined by Dipti Itchhaporia and published in the *Journal of the American College of Cardiology*, describes the evolution of the Triple Aim model over time [13]. I will briefly describe the intent of each aim and reframe each to demonstrate applicability to healthcare payers:

Patient Experience—The reality of healthcare in the United States is that it is a consumer driven practice. There are any number of reasons for this—political, historical, and societal— but there is not enough space to explore that topic fully here (if you are interested in learning more, I would recommend Dorothy Porter's *Health, Civilization and the State*). Patient experience dictates an individual's likelihood to engage in the health system [14] as well as their health literacy [15, 16] and the effectiveness of interventions [16, 17]. From a payer perspective, patient experience (or rather member experience) is far more existential. Member experience is a critical piece of a payer's value proposition. Plans that are difficult for patients to work with or, more simply, plans that do not pay enough attention to patient experience, see themselves out competed in the market space. My organization has a large, well-funded department focused on improving the member experience, not only with the organization but also with the providers within our network. Payers must work not only to improve the perception of health insurance companies (currently second only to cable providers in poor Net Promoter scores), but also to improve the perception of the health system as a whole. In many ways, they are the gateway and chief interaction point with the health system outside of the provider office or hospital room.

Quality of Care—The definition of quality of care is an amorphous and oftentimes shifting target, but the impact of "care quality" on the perceived value of care is not in question. Taking the consumerist viewpoint of healthcare into account, the outcomes of services that have been paid for are inherent to the theoretical model. Capitalism, in theory, seeks to maximize the quality of product or service for the most minimal cost possible. Consumers are—theoretically—incentivized to purchase health insurance plans that maximize their quality of care as a function of their willingness to pay increased insurance premiums based on the quality of care provided by the network to which those premiums grant them access. There is a great deal to unpack in that assertion, but before we descend too far into the foundations of capitalistic economics and their implications on the health insurance market, we'll return to "How do we define quality?" from the health insurance payer perspective. For this we will rely on Don Berwick himself. According to the IHI, Berwick defines quality of care as being comprised of six dimensions: "safety, effectiveness, patient-centeredness, timeliness, efficiency, and equity" [18]. From a traditional perspective, quality has been monitored by payers in direct response to maintenance of certifications or compliance with regulatory bodies.

More recently, there has been a broader recognition of the payer as an "integrator," a term coined and applied to payers by Berwick in the initial publication of the Triple Aim model [12]. In his perspective, payers should/must play a centralized role in the assurance of quality healthcare. Payers act as centralized data hubs (a concept covered in more detail later) as well as patient advocates arguing that care should be both affordable and as objectively high quality as possible. This shift has materialized in the "Value Transformation" movement. For the moment it will suffice to say that payers are waking up to their role in delivering quality care as defined above, but further transformation is needed to fully recognize their potential.

Cost of Care—The measurement of cost of care has been the most contentious of the original triple aim objectives. Providers and payors fundamentally disagree with the mechanisms that are available to control costs. For one, providers reimbursed under a fee-for-service model, faced with mounting economic pressures, are disincentivized from curbing medical expenditures. Payers have long been accused (rightly, in many cases) of seeking to curb medical costs merely to improve profit margins, but at its core the payer argument for controlling cost of care is this—good-quality care should be provisioned with as little expenditure as possible. With the classic "three-legged stool" model of health systems in mind, it is easy to see where the incentives for managing this aim lie. Providers, in the fee-for-service model, are incentivized to manage costs, insofar as the inflation of cost for the procedures and services provided does not exceed the price elasticity of the payor's willingness to pay for those services. Patients are conversely motivated to identify

> **Providers and payors fundamentally disagree with the mechanisms that are available to control costs.**

and utilize services at the lowest attainable price. This is simplistic reasoning, though, as patients rarely have the intricate knowledge necessary to advocate for their best interests, either in the election of treatments or the intricacies of the US medical billing system. This puts the individual patient at a distinct disadvantage in their effort to manage medical costs. These two unbalanced legs, I would argue, inform the need for insurers in the US, though they rarely advertise this service in their value proposals.

Insurers, with their margin motives and teams of medical professionals on staff, are the only constituent of the three-legged model that have both the incentive and specialized medical knowledge to manage this aim appropriately. One could argue they have attempted to play this role for the better part of a century with middling success. I would argue that this lack of success is a result of their singular focus, ignoring the other aims and the impact of these aims on the value proposition of healthcare. I would additionally argue that payers must understand and accept this adjustment of their mission: not only should they control costs, but they must also take an active role in the creation of healthcare value.

Provider Access/Retention—Contrary to Cost of Care, the fourth aim added to the quadruple aim has not been embraced by payers, but there is a clear reality that they must understand and embrace in order to transform the health system. The "product" that insurance companies sell is preferred access to a list of providers; in the industry, this is known as the "provider network." This network relies on the availability of a diverse set of provider specialties to achieve Centers for Medicare and Medicaid Services (CMS) mandated adequacy targets (geographic/demographic targets for representation by specialty). Historically, greater diversity/competition among provider groups has translated to improved cost and quality for patients in a given area. However, the trends of economic unsustainability in the provision of medical care have put exceedingly greater pressures on medical providers, particularly independent providers. This in turn has led to trends of practice closures and system consolidations that has reduced 1) the diversity of practice selection and 2) the reduction in specialty adequacy across the country. And this was all before COVID. We are just now beginning to recognize the impact of provider attrition resulting from the pandemic. The implications of these changes are clear: provider access and availability can no longer just be the concern of provider interest groups and traditional public health institutions (State Boards).

If current trends in the provider availability continue, payers face two catastrophic outcomes: 1) rural network adequacy will plummet, reducing the value proposition for providing health insurance in rural settings 2) consolidation in metropolitan areas will increase prices to the point where payers will no longer be able to charge premiums that enrollees can afford.

If current trends in the provider availability continue, payers face two catastrophic outcomes: 1) rural network adequacy will plummet, reducing the value proposition for providing health insurance in rural settings, and 2) consolidation in metropolitan areas will increase prices to the point where payers will no longer be able to charge premiums that enrollees can afford. Put simply, payers need a robust and healthy provider ecosystem to sustain their product. They must proactively engage with the provider community (and training pipeline) to ensure sustainability of the community. In extreme cases, this may mean sacrificing margin to meet sustainability goals in underserved regions. Failure to do so risks collapse of both the health system in a given area and the payer's health plan.

Health Equity—The final aim represents an industry wide revolution and epiphany that health doesn't begin with disease. The burgeoning field of the Social Determinants of Health (SDoH) and the recognition that provision and experience of care have not been equal across racial, ethnicity, primary spoken language (REL), sexual orientation, and gender identity lines has awoken both providers and payers to their roles in improving patient experiences. Providers, particularly those serving areas of lower socio-economic status (SES) or with higher proportions of racial and ethnic minority populations, have augmented community outreach and coalition work. Some payers, similarly, have embraced this call to action by either participating in community health coalitions or forming distinct partnerships. For both parties, however, this activity has focused on near term wins (not to deprecate the value of the initiatives). Food insecurity has been a primary target for both groups. Transportation and housing have also been common targets. These are certainly worthy causes, but they are characterized by one simple fact: they deliver quick (if less transformative) results. Feeding hungry people very quickly [19-21] improves the health outcomes of those individuals, but it does little to ameliorate the long-term inequities that contribute to food insecurity.

Thornier issues like safe, affordable living conditions and generational education are deemed to be outside of the purview of payer and provider alike. This is short sighted. As one of my doctoral cohort peers often explained, healthcare expenditures in the US exceed all other developed economies by a wide margin [22], but when social service spending is added, the US stands in a much less stark position (Figure 2) [23].

Figure 2: Total Health-service and Social-services Expenditures for Organization for Economic Co-operation and Development (OECD) Countries, 2005

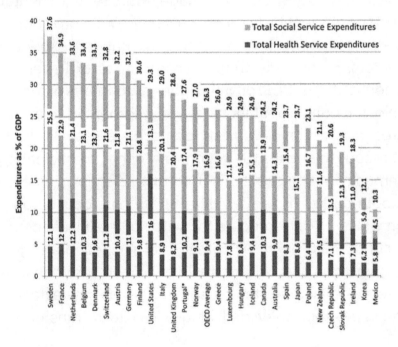

The reality is the United States pays for poor health outcomes in an acute setting. If we were to invest in preventative-transformative social services, we would avert much of this spending. As mentioned earlier in the motives section, few organizations are more compelled to reduce the cost burden of healthcare than payers, but the answer to those causes is long-term investments in community improvement. Payers must realize this role (either as conveners or leaders) to ensure the health systems sustainability and their own long-term viability.

> The reality is the United States pays for poor health outcomes in an acute setting. If we were to invest in preventative-transformative social services, we would avert much of this spending.

Information Integrators

As a data and analytics professional, I would be remiss if I did not at least mention the role of information in the transformation of the payer's role in population health. In some ways this argument will borrow from Berwick's argument for payers to serve the role of "integrator." Payers have a unique position within the health system: for all intents and purposes, any activity within the health system, that hopes to be reimbursed for its services, must submit information to the patient's health insurer. The patients themselves, apart from specific exclusions established by PPACA (aka ACA or "Obamacare"), are often required to submit information to the insurer on prior disease conditions and health in order to be underwritten for insurance. Large groups ensuring themselves under the Employee Retirement Income Security Act (ERISA aka Administrative

Services Only, ASO, or Self-Insured Organizations) usually contract with payers to gain access to their networks and to access their medical or pharmacy claims processing services. The net effect of this activity is a wealth of data—the raw material of the modern age—concentrated at the payer's disposal. Increasingly this data is integrated with additional consumer preference data (payers have extensive sales operations) and even credit information gathered as part of the application process, which supplements the medical history data available from the individual's claims experience. Partnerships with community organizations and federal/state/local governments provide enriched data on SDoH and Health Equity concerns. Altogether the data available to many insurers mesmerize most epidemiologists and it far surpasses most public health datasets in both breadth and depth.

This, however, is the briefest glimpse of the iceberg's tip. Data in and of itself has little applicable value: there is a reason we have coined this the "information age" not the "data age." Information requires dedicated teams of analytics professionals. Artificial Intelligence and Machine Learning professionals (often called Data Scientists), statisticians, and, yes, even epidemiologists often find employment in the payer space. These professionals turn this raw data material into information and knowledge. This is a key role that payers play

> **Not only is this data instrumental in the improvement of health systems operations—for example, identifying patients with key engagement opportunities associated with value based care arrangements—but also filling a key public health data availability gap.**

in the new world of population health. Not only is this data instrumental in the improvement of health systems operations—for example, identifying patients with key engagement opportunities associated with value based care arrangements—but also filling a key public health data availability gap. The public health publication space is replete with information about the publicly insured (Medicare and Medicaid), but our academic information on those individually covered or covered by ESI is quite limited. As mentioned above, this is the majority of the population. Payers must recognize the population health and public health role that they can play by making this information available to the academic and policy sphere.

Redefining Roles

In this chapter, I have outlined the motives and capabilities of payers in the health system. Now, I believe it is time to layout the strategic framework to realize this opportunity.

Payers as architects and arbiters of the redefinition of the value proposition of healthcare. I have laid out that payers are simultaneously uniquely economically incented and capacitated to advocate for all five of the quintuple aims. Their unique existential reliance on all five aims creates a pressing need to engage in improvements in the health system. Their central position as financiers of healthcare ensures that they have relationships established to enact change. Their comparative resources—both monetary, technological, and human capital—give them unique abilities to serve in a central role.

Payers as stewards of population health. Given their broad representation of the population of the country, payers can and should embrace their role as population health leaders. This behavior is in the payer's best interests from a business perspective because consumers seek services that are more than just claims processors and appreciable advancement of population health positively impacts the payer's bottom line.

Payers as sources of information for health innovation. Their unique data access and retention enables in-depth studies of populations not often available through traditional study datasets. Their relationships enable action at systemic scales. Combining these two elements, data and relationships, would drive key innovations in health care, population health, and society as a whole.

I am under no illusions: this shift in position and relationship requires significant investment and will be met with both skepticism and resistance from all players in the health system. However, I believe now more than ever, we are united by a common fate. COVID has revealed the weaknesses inherent in our health system. As of this writing, inflation looks to drive the US into recession. In short, we (the members of the health system) can no longer see ourselves as individual combatants. There are existential threats that will take each of us down individually if we do not unite against them.

> However, I believe now more than ever, we are united by a common fate.

References:

1) Kaiser Family Foundation. Health insurance coverage of the total population. 2021. Accessed November 5, 2022. https://www.kff.org/other/state-indicator/total-population/?currentTimeframe=0&sortModel=%7B%22colId%22:%22Location%22,%22sort%22:%22asc%22%7D.

2) Kaiser Family Foundation. Total Medicaid MCO enrollment. 2020. Accessed November 5, 2022. https://www.kff.org/other/state-indicator/total-medicaid-mco-enrollment/?currentTimeframe=0&sortModel=%7B%22colId%22:%22Location%22,%22sort%22:%22asc%22%7D.

3) Tarazi W, Welch P, Nguyen N, Bosworth A, Sheingold S, De Lew N, Sommers BD. Medicare beneficiary enrollment trends and demographic characteristics. U.S. Department of Health and Human Services, Office of the Assistant Secretary for Planning and Evaluation website. Published March 2, 2022. Accessed November 5, 2022. https://aspe.hhs.gov/reports/medicare-enrollment.

4) Hinton E, Stolyar L. 10 things to know about Medicaid managed care. Kaiser Family Foundation website. Published February 23, 2022. Accessed November 5, 2022. https://www.kff.org/medicaid/issue-brief/10-things-to-know-about-medicaid-managed-care/.

5) Freed M, Fuglesten B, Damico A, Neuman T. Medicare
    Advantage in 2022: Enrollment update and key trends. Kaiser
    Family Foundation website. Published August 25, 2022.
    Accessed November 5, 2022.
    https://www.kff.org/medicare/issue-brief/medicare-
    advantage-in-2022-enrollment-update-and-key-trends/.

6) National Association of Insurance Commissioners. U.S. health
    insurance industry analysis report. NAIC website. Updated
    July 21, 2022. Accessed November 5, 2022.
    https://content.naic.org/sites/default/files/inline-
    files/health-2022-mid-year-industry-report.pdf.

7) McKillop M, Liebermann D. The impact of chronic
    underfunding on America's public health system: trends,
    risks, and recommendations, 2022. Trust for America's Health
    website. Published July 2022. Accessed November 5, 2022.
    https://www.tfah.org/wp-
    content/uploads/2022/07/2022PublicHealthFundingFINAL.
    pdf.

8) Kirchhoff S. *Medical Loss Ratio Requirements under the
    Patient Protection and Affordable Care Act (ACA): Issues for
    Congress.* Congressional Research Service; 2018.

9) Morrisey M. *Health Insurance.* Second edition. AUPHA/HAP;
    2020.

10) Porter, D. *Health, Civilization and the State: A History of
    Public Health from Ancient to Modern Times.* Routlage; 1999.

11) Nundy S, Cooper LA, Mate KS. The quintuple aim for health care improvement: A new imperative to advance health equity. *JAMA*. 2022;327(6):521–522. doi:10.1001/jama.2021.25181.

12) Berwick DM, Nolan TW, Whittington J. The triple aim: care, health, and cost. *Health Aff.* 2008;27(3):759–769. doi: 10.1377/hlthaff.27.3.759.

13) Itchhaporia D. The evolution of the quintuple aim: Health equity, health outcomes, and the economy. *J. Am. Coll. Cardiol.* 2021;78(22):2262–2264. doi: 10.1016/j.jacc.2021.10.018.

14) Navarro S, Ochoa CY, Chan E, Du S, Farias AJ. Will improvements in patient experience with care impact clinical and quality of care outcomes?: A systematic review. *Med. Care.* 2021;59:843–856. doi:10.1097/mlr.0000000000001598.

15) Holden CE, Wheelwright S, Harle A, Wagland R. The role of health literacy in cancer care: A mixed studies systematic review. *PLoS One.* 2021;16(11):e0259815. doi: 10.1371/journal.pone.0259815.

16) Sepucha K, Atlas SJ, Chang Y, Dorrwachter J, Freiberg A, Mangla M, Rubash HE, Simmons LH, Cha T. Patient decision aids improve decision quality and patient experience and reduce surgical rates in routine orthopaedic care: A prospective cohort study. *J. Bone Joint Surg. Am.* 2017;99(15):1253–1260.

17) Poncelet AN, Hudson JN. Student continuity with patients: A system delivery innovation to benefit patient care and learning (continuity patient benefit). *Healthcare.* 2015;3(3):607–618. doi: 10.3390/healthcare3030607.

18) Berwick D. How can we define "quality" in health care? IHI website. Published Oct 21, 2008. Accessed November 5, 2022. https://www.ihi.org/education/IHIOpenSchool/resources/Pages/Activities/DefiningQualityAimingforaBetterHealthCareSystem.aspx.

19) Izumi BT, Martin A, Garvin T, Higgins Tejera C, Ness S, Pranian K, Lubowicki L. CSA partnerships for health: Outcome evaluation results from a subsidized community-supported agriculture program to connect safety-net clinic patients with farms to improve dietary behaviors, food security, and overall health. *Transl Behav Med.* 2020;10:1277–1285.

20) Cook M, Ward R, Newman T, Berney S, Slagel N, Bussey-Jones J, Schmidt S, Lee JS, Webb-Girard A. Food security and clinical outcomes of the 2017 Georgia fruit and vegetable prescription program. *J Nutr Educ Behav.* 2021;53(9):770–778. doi: 10.1016/j.jneb.2021.06.010.

21) Rivera RL, Maulding MK, Eicher-Miller HA. Effect of Supplemental Nutrition Assistance Program-Education (SNAP-Ed) on food security and dietary outcomes. *Nutr. Rev.* 2019;77(12):903–921. doi: 10.1093/nutrit/nuz013.

22) Organisation for Economic Cooperation and Development (OECD). Health at a glance 2019: OECD indicators. OECD iLibrary. Published 2019. Accessed November 5, 2022. https://www.oecd-ilibrary.org/sites/4dd50c09-en/index.html?itemId=/content/publication/4dd50c09-en.

23) Bradley EH, Elkins BR, Herrin J, Elbel B. Health and social services expenditures: Associations with health outcomes. BMJ Qual. Saf. 2011;20(10):826–831. doi: 10.1136/bmjqs.2010.048363.

Call to Action

THIS BOOK IS not an end, it is a continuation of improving the systems we are developing, research we are conducting, programs we are implementing, leaders we are training, and means by which we are evaluating our success in driving health for those counting on us.

At a minimum, if you continue to pursue your area of expertise and impact, please consider how it fits into the bigger picture of health—not just for you but for those you serve.

If you are a **medical scientist**, please consider how your expertise and tools can be or are complimented by public health science. As you continuously improve, what are your outcomes and data telling you? See the community face made up from all of the patients and families you are treating. Should things stay the same or are there key areas to do things differently? Is there an opportunity to find the common ground and force multiply? Join treatment and prevention tools to prescribe with rigor?

If you are a **public health scientist**, please consider how your expertise and tools can be complimented by medical science. As you continuously improve, what are your outcomes and data telling you? See the individual face in your communities you are serving. Should things stay the same or are there key areas to do things differently? Is there an opportunity to find the common ground and force multiply? Join treatment and prevention tools to prescribe with rigor?

If you are a **community leader**, consider how you impact health and healthcare, what tools you provide or need to drive health in your community.

If you are a **nonprofit leader**, consider how you fit into the fabric of solutions, including the data you have, and the access points you provide.

If you are a **dean of a medical school, public health school, business school, healthcare administration school,** etc., consider how you help your students learn by cross pollinating the education process and aligning measures of success on a broader scale.

If you are a **tech company leader**, consider how your data sets, predictive analytics, and AI look longitudinally and consider the expertise of a mix of scientists and economists so we learn all the data is telling us—not just the niche we are focused on.

If you are a **private equity investor**, consider funding to construct the new system and the major change, shifting the revenue and expense profile of health for America.

If you are an **integrated delivery network or payer**, consider the public health scientists value on your team, not just medical scientists.

If you are a **federal, state, or local government official**, please spend time aligning to the broader scoreboard and using the existing data to identify where the funding can make the most impact, including meaningful policy change. The data is there— use it please.

As an **individual and human**, consider the lifestyle you lead and identify one thing you can augment or change to help you achieve your health goals. If you need help to do it, our health system in America should be aligned to help you achieve your goals. We should be in this together. Are we?

To all of us, continue to improve together using outcome metrics at the macro and micro level—aligning the funding to the issues. Challenge the current traditional systems we consider best in class—are they really? Are we proactive or reactive? Is it built for the health of people and communities or is it built to support the business metrics and revenue projections?

The time is now—let's do it together.

Dr. Katie Kaney, DrPH, MBA, FACHE

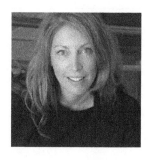

Dr. Katie Kaney is a C-suite healthcare thought leader with over 25 years of experience developing and implementing innovative programs to enhance care, promote health, and expand business models for success. She's the founder of The Whole Person Index, a former CAO for a large integrated delivery network, and a strategic advisor for multiple national and global companies. Kaney is a Fellow through the American College of Healthcare Executives, a lifelong community volunteer, and was named one of the Top 25 Women in Business in Charlotte, NC among numerous other accolades. Kaney earned her DrPH in Public Health and Health Leadership from UNC Gillings School of Global Public Health, and her MBA and BA from the University at Buffalo. **Both/And: Medicine and Public Health Together** is her first book. Learn more at:

www.WholePersonIndex.com

Printed in the USA
CPSIA information can be obtained
at www.ICGtesting.com
JSHW020225081024
71056JS00003B/14